VEINS

Everything You Need to Know

for Health and Beauty

VEINS

Everything You Need to Know
for Health and Beauty

Bridget F. Ostrow, M.D., F.A.C.S.
Louis B. Ostrow, M.D., F.A.C.S.

Doctors Book Press
Memphis, Tennessee

Published by:
Doctors Book Press
6209 Poplar, Suite 200
Memphis, Tennesse 38119
901-818-0100
www.theveincenter.com
lbostrow@theveincenter.com

ISBN: 0-9670025-3-2

PRINTED IN THE UNITED STATES OF AMERICA

Book Production: Phelps & Associates, Book Producers
Editors: Janice Phelps, Peter Bumpus
Cover Design: Frank Morris
Illustrations: Eddie Tucker

Environmental note: All printed materials used in this paperback have been produced with environmental considerations in mind.

Cataloging-in-Publication Data
(Provided by Quality Books, Inc.)

Ostrow, Bridget F.
    Veins : everything you need to know for
health and beauty / Bridget F. Ostrow & Louis B.
Ostrow. -- 1st ed.
    p. cm.
    Includes index
    ISBN: 0-9670025-3-2

    1. Veins--Diseases--Popular works.
I. Ostrow, Louis B.   II. Title

RC695.O78 1999   616.1'4
                    QBI99-101

Physicians' Profiles

Bridget F. Ostrow, M.D., director of The Vein Center in Memphis, Tennessee, is fully board certified in general surgery with special added qualifications in vascular surgery. She was one of the first women in the U.S. to be board certified in vascular surgery. Her medical degree was earned at St. Louis University, and she completed her internship, general surgery residency, and vascular surgery fellowship at the St. Louis University Hospitals. After completing her training, she was an assistant professor of surgery at St. Louis University and the University of Tennessee, Memphis. She is a fellow of the American College of Surgeons and a member of medical and surgical societies. She has received a number of medical and surgical awards.

Louis B. Ostrow, M.D., chief of surgery at The Vein Center in Memphis, Tennessee, is board certified in general surgery and thoracic surgery. He obtained his medical degree from the New York Medical College and completed his internship and general surgery residency at David Grant United States Air Force Medical Center, Travis Air Force Base, California. He also was the United States Air Force Trauma and Burn Fellow in the department of surgery at the University of California, San Francisco, General Hospital. He completed his cardiovascular and thoracic surgery training at the University of Tennessee, Memphis, and was formerly the chairman of cardiothoracic surgery at a regional medical center. He is a fellow of the American College of Surgeons and the American College of Chest Physicians. He also is the recipient of numerous medical and surgical awards.

To Anne, Rachel, Samuel, and Eli,
who make it all worthwhile.

Contents

FIGURE LEGENDS

Chapter 1

Figure 1. The Circulatory System of Your Body

Figure 2. The Greater Saphenous Vein

Figure 3. The Perforator Veins of the Calf

Figure 4. The Veins of Your Arm

Figure 5. One-way Vein Valves

Figure 6. Malfunctioning Valves Leading to Varicose Veins

Figure 7. The Calf Muscles Squeeze Blood Out of the Leg

Figure 8. Blood Flow Patterns in Leg Veins

Chapter 3

Figure 1. Spider Veins Before and After Treatment

Figure 2. How Sclerotherapy Works

Figure 3. How Lasers and Pulsed-light Therapy Works

Chapter 4

Figure 1. Varicose Veins Before and After Treatment

Figure 2. Malfunctioning Valves Leading to Varicose Veins

Chapter 5

Figure 1. Facial Spider Veins Before and After Treatment

Chapter 6

Figure 1. Superficial Thrombophlebitis

Figure 2. Deep Vein Thrombosis

Figure 3. Blood Clot Lodged in the Pulmonary Artery

Chapter 7

Figure 1. Hyperpigmentation of the Leg

Figure 2. Open Venous Ulcer in a Patient Whose Only Risk Factor Was
Untreated Varicose Veins

Chapter 8

Figure 1. A Clot Forming in an Arm Vein Surrounding a Catheter

Figure 2. The First Rib Causing Arm Vein Obstruction

Foreword

As a vein treatment specialist, I deal firsthand with the lack of accurate information available regarding vein problems at both the patient and physician level.

Antiquated techniques for both varicose and spider vein treatment have kept costs high and satisfaction low. The use of lasers has now found its place in the treatment of spider veins allowing a "no needles" method of ridding this cosmetically dissatisfying condition. With the development of office-based varicose vein surgery, which along with Drs. Ostrow I have helped pioneer, patients can return to work and a normal lifestyle the next day at a fraction of the expense and discomfort previously encounter when treating these problems.

This book, *Veins: Everything You Need to Know for Health and Beauty*, gives up-to-the-minute approaches to the vein problems we commonly see. It gives an overview of the condition and the therapies we, as dedicated vein care specialists, would expect to work.

In summary, everyone that has or treats vein problems, physicians and patients alike, should read this book. It provides current teachings on what "those in the know" would recommend for these common but often misunderstood problems. I congratulate Drs. Ostrow on their effort.

Ronald G. Bush, M.D.
Director
Midwest Vein Treatment Clinics
Cincinnati Vein Center

Note to Our Readers

Acknowledgment

We would like to thank Sylvia Hall for her unending assistance in the preparation of multiple drafts of this book.

We would like to express our appreciation to patients we have had the privilege of caring for over our many years of training and practice. We would especially like to thank those who suffer with vein disorders. You were the motivation to write this book. You are indeed the "silent majority" in this country.

INTRODUCTION

These Are Real Problems!

"My legs look like road maps!"

You wake up one day and notice a few little blue lines on your thighs. You think nothing of it. Then you get some purple ones. Then a few red ones. With time it seems like they are covering every spot on your legs. You try to get a tan, maybe that will help. You try covering them with makeup, but you have to spend half an hour every morning just putting makeup on your legs. Then you stop wearing skirts.

Each day you look in the mirror to see if they're getting worse, and lo and behold, they *are* worse. You ask your spouse or a friend about them. They say, "They're no big deal. Almost everyone your age has them. All your friends at the pool have them." "Everyone your age has them." Is that supposed to make you feel better? What do you care about everyone else? This is driving you crazy!

So for years you go on, unhappy, embarrassed, and self-conscious. You won't wear shorts, skirts, or a bathing suit. After a while you finally get the nerve to ask your doctor what to do. You make an appointment, spend an hour in the waiting room, pay your money, and finally get to ask, "What can I do about these ugly spider veins?" He tells you, "Don't worry; it's just a cosmetic problem. Even my wife has them and they are worse than yours."

Now you're not worried, you're angry. It may be cosmetic to the rest of the world, but it's ruining your life. It limits what you do. It limits what you wear. It feels like a lot more than just cosmetics.

So you ask your girlfriend about the veins. She knew someone who had her veins injected by some doctor you've never heard of, but the needle sticks hurt and burned. In some places the veins came back worse than what she started with.

Now what do you do? Every few months a new blue highway seems to be forming on your legs.

*

"I won't wear shorts with these legs!"

You just had your second baby. She is beautiful! But during the last trimester of your pregnancy you started developing bulging veins on the inside of both your legs. They ached so much; sometimes you could hardly stand. Your obstetrician told you they were varicose veins and that they should go away shortly after the delivery. But now the baby is 4 months old and the veins are still there. They look like grape clusters hanging off your legs. Even your husband made a comment about them.

You go back and see your obstetrician again. She puts you in a paper gown, you lie down on the exam table, a little poking and prodding, and then you stand up. The veins bulge out and you start developing that aching sensation all the way down to your toes. She says, "Good news. It's only varicose veins. When you called, I was worried that something bad had happened. Lots of women have varicose veins. I'm starting to get them too. I wouldn't be too concerned. If they become a real problem, we can have a surgeon strip them out."

You think to yourself: *Great, am I the only one that takes this seriously? If I didn't think it already was a problem, I wouldn't be here. My mother had her veins stripped after my kid brother was born. To this day, she still tells horror stories about it. My grandmother had to come and help take care of us. My mother was in the hospital for 3 days, off work for 4 weeks and black-and-blue for 2 months. Now all I have to do is wait for my legs to get bad enough to have this done to me. In the meantime, I get to watch my legs get worse while I get more embarrassed. Besides, my legs still ache. Isn't there anything I can do?*

*

As physicians, we hear these stories each and every day. The details may change, but the plot stays the same. We're commonly told:

"I won't go to the swimming pool with my kids."

"I wear dark hose so people won't see my ugly legs."

"My legs throb all the time."

"My grandson pointed at my legs and said, 'Grandma, how did you hurt yourself?' "

You, too, may be saying these kinds of things on a daily basis. But you're not alone. Varicose and telangiectatic leg veins (better known as spider veins) occur in up to 80 million adults in the United States.[1] That's one third of the population. A 1972 United States Public Health Service survey reported that over 33% of all people in the United States had varicose veins. Three million of them are under the age of 45.[2] With over 20 million baby boomers reaching their early fifties by the turn of the century, and 1 baby boomer turning 50 every 7 seconds for the next 18 years, the numbers are astounding. Varicose veins occupy seventh place in incidence among 28 chronic diseases.[13] It has been estimated that at least 25% of all American women, young and old, have varicose veins. The percentage increases in older women. By the time they reach their seventies an estimated 72% of American women will have varicose veins.[3-5] This problem is not isolated to women, however. An estimated 42% of all Americans over 60 years old develop varicose veins,[3,4] and spider veins are just as common. Studies have demonstrated that 35% of the women in the United States and 10% of the men have this condition.[12]

Vein disorders are the most common blood vessel problem known to man.[9] They are 10 times more prevalent in this population than hardening of the arteries[10] and occur far more often than heart disease, our nation's number one killer. But they receive little attention in either the public or the medical press. This is unfortunate, because as a result most patients do not receive appropriate care for problems such as varicose veins until they develop complications.

Although it has long been believed by physicians and patients that varicose and spider veins are merely a cosmetic nuisance, over 50% of the patients who seek treatment do so because of pain and discomfort.[1] In addition, approximately 150,000 Americans die each year from vein-related complications. Over 2.5 million others have significant disabilities such as chronic venous insufficiency,[6,7] and at least 500,000 have chronic venous leg sores,[7] which is more than 1% of the U.S. population. All told, nearly 100,000 individuals are totally disabled by these conditions.[3] Most of those affected are women.

It has been estimated that in this country 2 million workdays are lost every year from venous leg sore complications.[11] If these ulcers had been treated properly, there would have been less pain and expense. Furthermore, if the patients had been treated prior to the onset of the open sores, far less pain and suffering would have occurred.

This is not just a problem in America. In Germany, more than 25% of the adult population show marked abnormalities in their leg veins, 15% have chronic venous insufficiency, and more than 1.2 million individuals suffer from chronic leg ulcers. It has been estimated that the cost of treating leg ulcers in Germany is DM 2.5 billion,[8] which is equivalent to about $1.4 billion U.S. dollars per year in a country less than half the size of the U.S. This doesn't even include the treatment of varicose or spider veins, the most common vein problems.

If all vein problems are considered, close to 45% of the people in the industrialized world are affected—close to 1 billion people. If developing nation populations are also included, a staggering 2 billion people may be affected.

This book will give you a better understanding of varicose veins and spider veins, and treatments and possible complications will be explored. We will also describe a host of other common and often misunderstood vein problems. We will try to dispel the misinformation circulating about these conditions and tell you the real story. You will get the facts! We believe that an informed patient can make rational choices regarding treatment of their vein disorders.

If you are one of the millions of women suffering with vein problems, take heart. An understanding of your condition and a discussion of possible solutions is just a few pages away. By drawing on illustrative cases from our extensive vein care practice, many possible solutions to a variety of conditions will come to light. But, perhaps the best news of all is— you're not alone!

CHAPTER 1

Understanding Your Circulation

"I have these veins that bulge out of my legs. Maybe it's a circulation problem? I know somebody that lost a leg. I wonder if that could happen to me?"

To discuss how veins function and malfunction in your body, a basic understanding of the circulatory system is needed. Almost 1 in every 7 Americans has a disease that involves some part of the blood vessel system. These malfunctions are responsible for 53% of all deaths in America.[1] Varicose veins are the most common blood vessel problem in this country.

To understand the circulatory system, a description of its various components is necessary. The heart is essential. It is the central organ necessary for the maintenance of life, beating approximately 70 times per minute throughout your life—faster in a child, slower in an adult. A blockage in one of the coronary arteries, the blood vessels that carry oxygenated blood to the heart itself, often leads to a heart attack and possibly death. This can occur either quickly or slowly. Indeed, heart disease is the leading cause of death in the United States.

There are four chambers in the heart, two pumping and two collecting. The right side of the heart collects blood from throughout the body, then pumps it to the lungs where it is oxygenated. The blood is then passed on to the left side of the heart, which pumps the blood to the remainder of the body. (Figure 1)

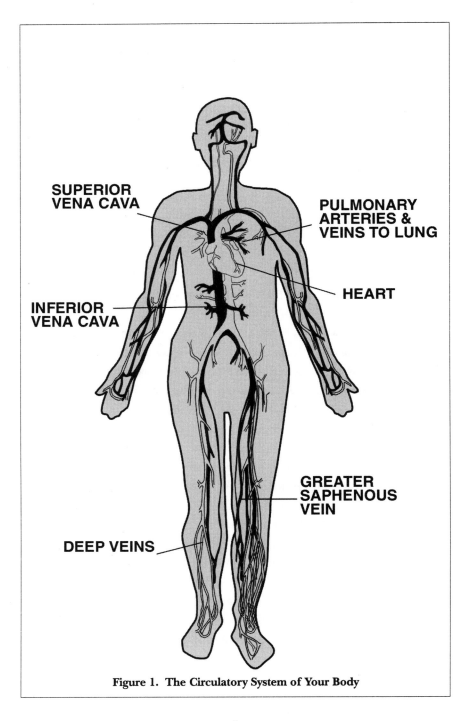

Figure 1. The Circulatory System of Your Body

Arteries carry oxygenated blood away from the heart, and blood flows through arteries at elevated pressures. When doctors or nurses take your blood pressure, they are measuring the pressure in the arteries.

The blood flows from larger arteries into smaller arteries, until it eventually reaches the nourishing capillary beds. These blood vessels are so small that red blood cells line up and move through them in single file. These vessels decrease the blood pressure that reaches the muscles and other organs. In the capillary beds, oxygen is exchanged for carbon dioxide and other waste products in the system. Once the blood leaves the capillary beds, it is called venous blood. Veins carry desaturated blood (low oxygen content blood) from the muscles and organs back to the heart. Small veins join together to form larger and larger veins that eventually become the two main veins to the heart, the superior and inferior venae cavae. This completes the round trip circuit of blood flow through the body.

Approximately 75% of all your body's blood is in the peripheral veins in your legs.[2] These act as a reservoir for supplying blood to wherever you need it, but the amount of blood in your legs varies with position. When you are standing, several pints of blood pool there.[4-5] When you are lying flat, the amount is less. This is why veins tend to bulge out of your legs when you stand. Any problem in your leg veins affects your whole body since most of your blood is stored there.

THE PROBLEM WITH VEINS

Due to their thin walls, veins are prone to malfunction,[3] and most vein problems occur in the legs. Two distinct vein systems run through the legs. A superficial set runs just under the skin called the saphenous veins. The deep veins are the other set.

The greater saphenous vein is the longest vein in the body, running from the ankle to the groin. At the level of the groin it joins up with the femoral vein, which is part of the deep venous system. The lesser saphenous vein runs along the back of your calves. It begins at the ankle and joins the popliteal vein of the deep vein system behind your knee. The saphenous veins are located in a layer of fat just below the skin. (Figure 2)

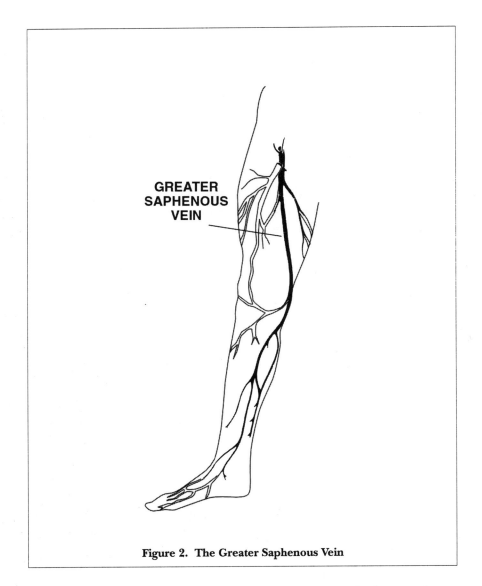

GREATER SAPHENOUS VEIN

Figure 2. The Greater Saphenous Vein

The deep veins run alongside the arteries near the bones of your leg surrounded by muscles and other connective tissue. Once the blood reaches the deep venous system in the leg, it travels from the femoral vein in your groin to the iliac vein in your pelvis and abdomen. These then join from each leg to form the inferior vena cava, which carries the blood back to the heart.

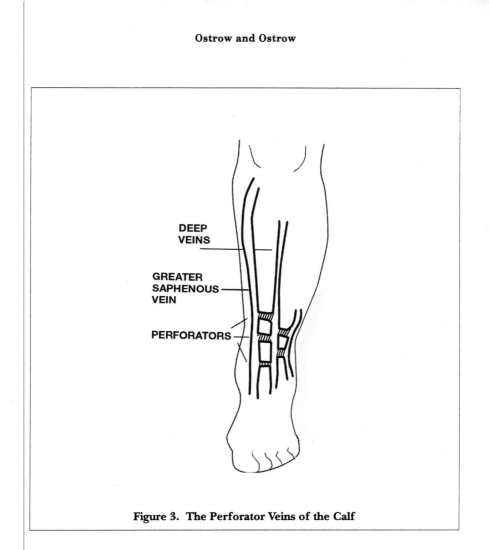

Figure 3. The Perforator Veins of the Calf

Perforator veins connect the saphenous and deep veins at different levels of the leg. (Figure 3) The number of perforator veins varies from person to person, from as few as 2 to as many as 6. Most of the perforator veins are located in the lower leg between the knee and ankle.

Arm veins are also found in superficial and deep groups. Much like in your legs, the superficial veins run right under the skin. Blood is drawn for laboratory tests from these veins, and intravenous catheters are inserted into them. The deep veins follow the arteries along the bones. Once the superficial and deep veins join, they course through your underarm (axilla) and shoulder to enter the chest. At this position they join to become the axillary vein. Under your collarbone the name

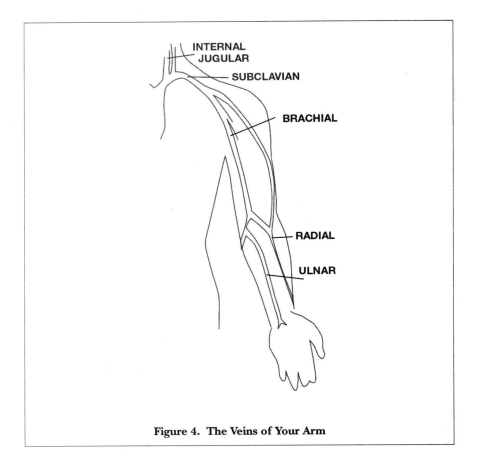

INTERNAL
JUGULAR

SUBCLAVIAN

BRACHIAL

RADIAL

ULNAR

Figure 4. The Veins of Your Arm

changes to the subclavian vein. In the chest this vein joins with those from the other arm and with the veins that drain blood from your head to form the superior vena cava. (Figure 4) This very large vein carries the blood from the upper part of the body back to your heart. In the arms, vein valves play a much less significant role in health and well-being than the valves in your legs.

ONE-WAY VALVES IN YOUR LEG VEINS

The valves in your veins act as one-way faucets that drive the blood back to your heart, making sure that the blood moves towards the heart and against the flow of gravity. (Figure 5) If these valves malfunction, varicosities or "abnormal" veins form. (Figure 6) The valves look like

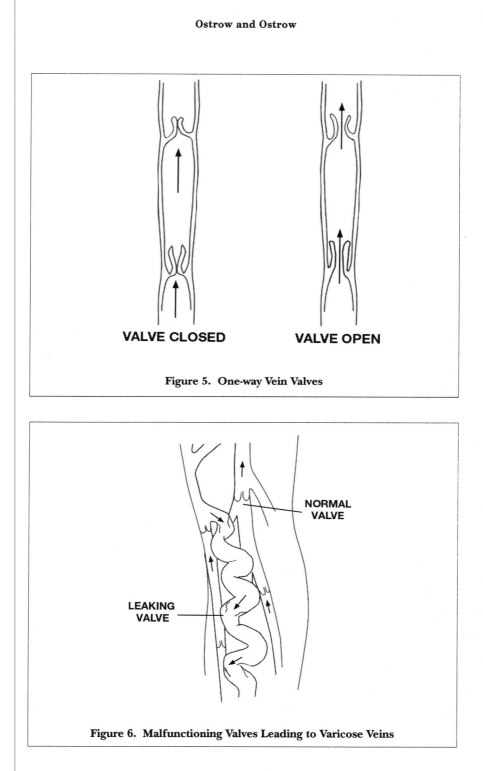

Figure 5. One-way Vein Valves

Figure 6. Malfunctioning Valves Leading to Varicose Veins

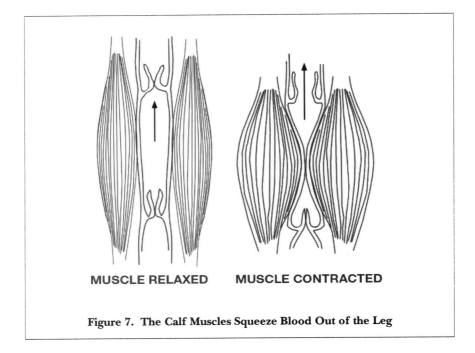

MUSCLE RELAXED   MUSCLE CONTRACTED

Figure 7. The Calf Muscles Squeeze Blood Out of the Leg

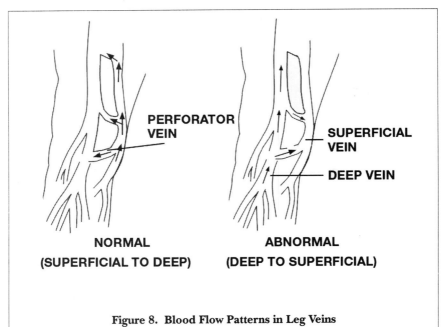

PERFORATOR VEIN

SUPERFICIAL VEIN

DEEP VEIN

NORMAL
(SUPERFICIAL TO DEEP)

ABNORMAL
(DEEP TO SUPERFICIAL)

Figure 8. Blood Flow Patterns in Leg Veins

little tissue-paper-thin parachutes that are attached to the sides of the vein wall. They are located at strategic points in blood vessels to insure that blood flows in the proper direction. Normally, when the valves are open, the blood flows in the direction of the heart, forced along the way by the muscles that surround the deep veins. As the muscles contract with exercise, walking, or normal movement, they squeeze the blood in the veins upward and back to the heart (Figure 7). If blood tries to flow the wrong way, the valves close tightly preventing blood from backing up in the system. Valves are also present in the perforator veins that control the flow of blood from the more superficial saphenous veins into the deep veins. When the vein valves fail, blood pools in the saphenous veins or flows in the reverse direction from the deep to the superficial saphenous veins. (Figure 8) With time, injury to the thin-walled saphenous veins occurs.

Vein valves can be injured and will subsequently fail for a variety of reasons. Direct injury to the vein as a result of trauma or a broken bone may cause a blood clot to develop that will cause the valve to take on an abnormal shape and no longer function. (This will be discussed in detail in a later chapter.) Also, obesity or extensive exercise can put abnormal pressure on a valve. In an attempt to control these problems, the body uses the valves to divide the legs into many individual compartments. Although the valve in one vein segment may not be working properly, the valves above and below it may be okay. Thus, localized rather than general problems usually occur. Because the leg veins bear your body's entire weight, they are the most prone to developing problems. The heavier you are, the more stress your leg veins are under, and the more difficult it is for the venous blood to flow uphill against gravity.

When someone develops problems in the deep system, blood is shunted through the perforator veins to the weaker superficial saphenous veins. This can cause the saphenous veins, which are not surrounded by strong muscles and connective tissue, to dilate, stretching open the one-way valves. As a result, further malfunctions may occur in the superficial system. There may be increased pressure that will allow blood and edema fluid to pool in your leg and leg veins, but more commonly, the saphenous veins, which are not protected and supported like the deep veins, are directly affected. They lose their shape, and they malfunction. Initially, the perforator veins can prevent the saphenous veins from becoming abnormally shaped because the perforator can be used as an escape route that allows blood to shift back and forth to the deep system. However, with time, this mechanism can fail and varicosities may form. Varicose veins have developed in almost 50% of all Americans by the time they reach their fifties.

SUMMARY

Blood flows through everyone's body in the same way. It is only due to disease or injury that significant variations occur. Scientists think a common reason for vein malfunction is their thin walls.

Valves in your leg veins help keep the blood flowing back to your heart. They prevent pooling of blood in your veins and legs. If the valves of the superficial veins malfunction, abnormal veins called varicosities form. Valve malfunction is associated with many of the problems discussed in later chapters.

Arm veins follow a similar pattern of deep and superficial systems, but in the arms, vein valves play a far less significant role than in the legs.

CHAPTER 2

You and Your Doctors

"I've got this dull ache in my calves. It's always worse at night. Sometimes it itches and burns."

Your legs have been hurting for months. The pain is worse when you stand; it seems to be a little better when you walk, but at night your legs really ache. Sometimes they even itch and burn. You thought the problem would go away on its own, but it hasn't. You tried different shoes, but that didn't help. Now you're worried you may have a circulation problem. Maybe you'll lose your leg? Maybe you'll need a big operation to save it? Each passing thought seems to make the discomfort worse.

When you see your family doctor, she says she doesn't see anything abnormal. She doubts it's a circulation problem, but she says to be on the safe side, you should see a surgeon. So you set up a consultation.

The surgeon says you have good pulses in your feet, it probably isn't an artery problem, and you won't lose your legs. But just to be sure he wants to order an ultrasound test to measure the blood flow. After all, you may have an unusual problem that he doesn't want to miss. You get the test done the following week at the hospital and then go back to the surgeon.

He says, "Good news, your circulation is okay! Nothing to worry about. I'm not sure what's causing your leg pain, but you should be fine. Maybe you should go back and see your family physician again."

And out of the office you go. Four weeks have passed since you called to make the original appointment with your primary care doctor. You now know your circulation is okay, so you're not going to lose your legs, but your calf discomfort is no better. They still ache every day. It's beginning to affect your life, and your husband is getting tired of hearing you complain about it every night! But what are you supposed to do? It still hurts. So you go back to your family doctor.

She's still not sure what is wrong. "Maybe you have a clot in the vein in your leg or maybe you have early diabetes, or maybe it's a nerve problem? It's not obvious, but we can't tell for sure without some tests," she says. So back to the hospital you go for another round of tests. Good news! No clots, no diabetes, no nerve problems. Bad news! Your legs still hurt every day and no one seems to be sure what's causing the problem.

At this point you are really disgusted. You've spent weeks and plenty of money running around, and you still have the same problem. Then, your family physician thinks of one more person you might try to see. A new vein center has opened. She's not sure they can help, but at this stage it can't hurt. So off you go to yet another doctor....

*

Half the problem with vein disorders is knowing where to go for treatment. A myriad of people can be involved with your care before you reach the right person. Many of those individuals may have little experience in dealing with complex vein conditions. Furthermore, physicians and surgeons often take different approaches to the same problem. Even specialists within the same field may vary in their treatment of these problems.

Unfortunately, with many vein conditions, there are no straightforward answers. Therapies may vary depending on the understanding of the problem, the treatment alternatives, the experience of the physician with this particular problem, and a sound plan the patient can agree to. Often, many of the approaches require a significant amount of patient involvement. For this reason a mutually agreed upon plan is important.

If you find that your current physician is not helping you through your problems, or does not have the level of expertise that you desire, we have some suggestions that may better serve your needs. Also remember, you are not alone. Millions of other people have the same problems and concerns. Vein problems need to be taken seriously, even if it takes some work on your part to find the help that is right for you.

HOW DO YOU KNOW WHEN A DOCTOR IS RIGHT FOR YOU?

Hopefully, you are satisfied with your present physicians. They should understand your medical problem and your concerns. In addition, there are certain things that all patients with vein problems should expect from a physician:

1. Is the doctor listening to you?

In medical school physicians are taught that the medical history gives 80% of the diagnosis. As doctors gain experience, however, they tend to listen less and less to their patients. Be sure that your physician listens and understands what you say.

2. Does your doctor examine you?

In the hurried world we live in, doctors can sometimes forget to take their time, but they must listen to their patients and examine them as well. When patients come back for frequent problems, such as open leg sores, it is all too easy to simply assume that nothing has changed. But in the case of vein problems it is critical that your doctors or any other health care professionals reevaluate your problem each and every time they see you.

3. Are you being treated with respect?

The doctor needs to let you explain your concerns about both your problem and the treatment. You should not be dismissed or ignored. After all, they are your problems, not your doctor's. The doctor's main role is to find a way to make you better. If you are unclear or dissatisfied, you need to let him or her know.

4. Are you getting enough information?

Your doctors should take enough time to explain your problem to you in detail, including the reasons why you have this problem and the various treatment alternatives available. Then in a language that you can understand, they should explain their reasons for suggesting one particular path over another. If they can't do this, or you if you don't understand them, ask questions. You should always leave the doctor's office understanding exactly what you are doing and why. If you don't, both you and your doctor are remiss.

5. Is your doctor treating you or your problem?

Frequently medical professionals hone in on fixing only the problem at hand. Doctors sometimes treat the problem and not the patient. In many cases lifestyle changes are needed to effect good long-term results. A more holistic approach is often necessary.

6. Can you reach your doctor?

Has your doctor gone over with you what to expect after your treatments? Is he readily available when you need him for an office appointment or on the telephone? Even though the doctor may not be able to speak directly with you, is a knowledgeable staff member such as a nurse, technician, or physician's assistant available to attend promptly to your needs? If the answer to this question is yes, then you can probably work through the other details. If the answer to this question is no, then you need to think about looking for another caregiver.

7. Are you a partner in your treatment?

Vein problems are complex. Your input is necessary, and it should be welcomed. When you are not able to play a role in making decisions, you often will not follow them. You must work together with your doctor to come up with the right plan for rectifying your problems.

THE DOCTORS YOU WILL MEET

There is no licensing body that regulates who can call themselves a vein specialist. Be aware that many people with different levels of expertise lay claim to the title. Fortunately, you often don't even need specialized care for vein problems; your primary health care providers

14

will be able to manage them. When they can't, they can often direct you to an individual with the appropriate level of training and expertise. The following is a list of physicians that you may encounter, as well as some information to help you select the physician right for you:

1. Primary Care Physicians: These individuals can manage many of your vein problems. Internists, general practitioners, family physicians, and gynecologists are likely to develop a long-term medical relationship with you. In addition, if they are treating you for other medical problems, they will already know much of your history. Many of them will have extensive experience with vein problems and will be able to relate them to other conditions you may have. The disadvantage to using these physicians is that some may lack the specialized knowledge often needed for difficult problems. Furthermore, many don't have the technical skills necessary to aggressively treat problems such as spider veins, varicose veins, and venous ulcers.

2. Specialists: There are a host of specialists experienced in treating different facets of vein problems, including dermatologists, general surgeons, plastic surgeons, cardiovascular surgeons, and vascular surgeons. These individuals will have varied experience and different approaches to treating individual problems, based on their background.

3. Vein Treatment Specialists: These are usually dermatologists or surgeons who specialize in the diagnosis and treatment of venous disease. These physicians often know the best and most cost-effective way to treat you. They are usually well-versed in all facets of vein disease and can offer various approaches for treatment. As an extension to this, vein centers are opening throughout the country staffed by individuals who have a bona fide interest in these problems. Many physicians are now limiting their practice to vein problems—just be sure that you choose physicians who have the expertise and the ability they claim to have. Since there currently is no credentialing process for becoming a vein specialist, anyone can use the title. Also, the approach of some specialists may not suit your individual needs, so be sure that you and your doctor can agree on a treatment plan before you commit to any approach.

HOW TO PICK A DOCTOR

You know your problem and the kind of individual that you want treating it, but how do you find that certain doctor? Often this takes time and effort.

Speaking with your own doctor will often direct you to the next appropriate level of care. Your friends and neighbors can also steer you in the proper direction. With 80 million individuals in the United States suffering with vein problems, everyone knows someone who has been treated. The odds are overwhelming that your friends can recommend several doctors in addition to those you already know.

Other organizations such as those listed at the end of this book can provide information regarding physicians and other vein treatment specialists in your area dedicated to these problems. The local county medical society is also a good source of information for doctors in your town. Many physicians now also offer this information on the internet. Our web site, for example, is **www.theveincenter.com.**

YOUR INITIAL CONSULTATION

At The Vein Center in Memphis, patients generally spend up to one hour in the office on their first visit. This includes taking a history, doing a physical examination with an emphasis on the venous system, explaining our approach to the particular problem, and a discussion about alternative care paths. Finally, we develop an agreeable treatment plan. Although this can be done in less time, we find that up to an hour can be required to discuss all the options and answer all of the questions.

THE HISTORY

We ask our patients about any medications that they are presently taking, any allergies to medications, their past medical and surgical history, their family's medical history, and what physical activities they are currently engaged in such as jogging and aerobics. We also want to know what other treatment modalities have been used for their problems. Some people find it helpful to write this information down prior to their initial visit.

It is especially important to document what medication you have taken, in what dosages, and when they were prescribed. Although vein problems generally do not require long-term prescription drugs, substances such as antibiotics and other associated medications may influence the treatment approach taken. Some drugs are photosensitive and can cause bad reactions during certain laser and light-based treatment plans.

Family history is also useful for understanding many problems. Heredity plays an important role in spider vein and varicose vein problems. In other problems such as blood clots, it is less relevant, unless certain familial biochemical abnormalities are present. Be concerned if a physician does not seem interested in your family history. They may be ignoring important information that can speed your diagnosis and treatment.

The history of your vein problem is especially important for developing a treatment plan. The patients' level of expectation and the satisfaction they can obtain frequently depend on how long a problem has been present and what has already been done. This information tells us what may or may not have worked in the past.

Some of the questions that should be asked are:
1. What is the primary problem?
2. When did your vein problem first develop? Was there an associated pregnancy or injury? Did you just start hormones or birth control pills?
3. Is the problem getting worse, or has it stayed the same?
4. Is this predominantly an appearance problem, or does it have physical symptoms?
5. Is there anyone else in your immediate family with this problem (parents, grandparents, sisters, or brothers)?
6. Is the problem worse on one leg?
7. Can you describe the sensation associated with the problem? For example, if there is pain present, is it throbbing or pounding or just aching?
8. How often do the symptoms occur? Are they related to your menstrual cycle? Are they dependent on the time of day? Do they occur with prolonged standing?

9. If there is discomfort, what makes it better?
10. What has and has not worked in the past to treat the problem?
11. Are you receiving ongoing treatment at this time? Are you sticking to the recommendations and schedule?
12. Is the problem interfering with your lifestyle?
13. Who has been overseeing the treatment of this problem in the past? Was it your primary care physician?
14. Have you been happy with your previous treatments?
15. Are there major life crises occurring that could affect the care and treatment of the problem?

By asking detailed questions, a physician can usually sort through the previous treatment approaches and find out whether some were more successful than others. In some cases, your current treatment may be the best. Or, this may be the first time you have sought treatment. All of these factors will impact your treatment plan.

REVIEW OF SYSTEMS

We ask general questions regarding other medical conditions on a system-by-system basis. We specifically ask about things such as high blood pressure, heart disease, ulcers, strokes, and bleeding disorders. These problems and their medications may adversely affect or contribute to vein and leg problems.

THE PHYSICAL EXAMINATION

Your doctor should give you a complete physical examination at the initial consultation. This will give him a better understanding of your general health status and tell him whether the problem is isolated or part of a larger medical condition. This will impact the therapeutic alternative chosen. For example, some of the elements in our initial physical examination are:

1. Vital signs: We measure the temperature, pulse rate, blood pressure, height, and weight.

2. Heart and Lungs: We listen for breath sounds as well as for heart murmurs, which gives us clues about the overall health of the patient.

3. Breasts: We ask each woman if she has any abnormal lumps or bumps in her breasts. We also ask if she has had a recent breast examination. When there is any concern or suspicion, we proceed with our own breast examination at this time.

4. Abdomen: We palpate for abnormal masses to make sure there is not an unrecognized cause for her problems.

5. Arteries: We feel the pulses to check for vascular problems. We also listen to the flow of blood through various neck arteries to check for abnormalities. We specifically check for the presence of pulses in the feet. If they are absent, it may impact therapeutic alternatives.

6. Legs: We examine the patient while she is lying down and standing, looking for spider veins, varicose veins, swelling, and open leg sores. We also look for associated skin changes.

DISCUSSING THE PROBLEM

At the end of the initial consultation we feel that it is important for a doctor to sit down with the patient and review his or her interpretation of the problem and all treatment alternatives. We then suggest a treatment plan customized for each individual patient. The consultation should include the following steps:

1. Discussing the main problem.
2. Reviewing the methods that have previously been used to treat a problem and why they may or may not have worked.
3. Discussing the best alternatives for treating the problem.
4. Discussing the pro's and con's of each treatment alternative.
5. Explaining the reasons for selecting a specific treatment plan.

We explain to our patients that in our opinion vein problems are not solely a cosmetic disorder. There are many physical problems associated with venous conditions that deserve treatment just as much as diabetes or heart disease.

We review the patient's expectations about their treatment. Some people want a "cure" for their problem. Others are satisfied if they are just a little better. Each person has a different level of expectation, but only through discussion can we discover what that level is. With some problems patients must be willing to participate to effect a good result. When patients are not eager to help with their own treatment, their physicians may need to select a different approach.

Occasionally other tests are needed before a final diagnosis can be given. This usually entails the use of ultrasound to give us a better look at the veins and their working parts. Other tests are seldom required.

Finally, you, the patient, should ask all of your questions. You should always leave the doctor's office satisfied that you understand the problem and its proposed therapy. Some of the questions that you may consider include:

1. Is this an unusual problem?
2. Have you treated many people with my condition?
3. What do you think is the cause of this condition?
4. How effective do you think the treatment plan will be?
5. How long will the treatment plan take?
6. What is the projected cost of this treatment?
7. What are my responsibilities in this treatment plan?

Some other thoughts to ponder are:

1. Does the doctor take my problem seriously? Does this person think that this is just a cosmetic nuisance or a true medical condition?
2. Is the physician interested in working with me to obtain the best treatment plan, or does he or she rubber stamp one treatment approach for everyone?
3. Did this person explain the problem and treatment well enough for me to understand them?
4. Does this person have a positive attitude about making my problem better?
5. Can I reach this person if a problem arises?
6. If this treatment plan does not work, does this person seem willing to help me find one that will?
7. Is the cost of the treatment in my budget?

If the answer to the majority of those questions is yes, then you will most likely want to proceed with care and treatment by this physician. Then it is up to the two of you to work together and agree on an approach that suits your needs. We generally try to start treatment at the first visit. We find that phone calls following each visit are an important part of vein treatment. Concerns or questions may pop up following the visit that can frequently be rectified with a brief conversation. This service is generally performed by our nurses. When an unusual question or problem arises, a verbal consultation with the physician is obtained. Patients should not have to wait until their next visit to alleviate concerns.

FOLLOW-UP VISITS

Most vein problems require more than one visit to the doctor. Spider veins may require 4 to 6 visits; varicose veins about the same, depending on the approach selected; leg ulcers more. The frequency and timing of the visits depend on the treatment path taken as well as the results obtained. Our first follow-up visit often occurs within 1 to 3 weeks of the initial visit or consultation.

THE ONGOING DOCTOR-PATIENT RELATIONSHIP

You have picked a doctor, seen him in consultation, and agreed on a treatment plan. An ongoing relationship has been established. Some relationships may last only weeks, others may be lifelong. The situation with each individual is different; however, both the patient and the doctor always have certain responsibilities.

The doctor's responsibilities include:

1. Keeping up to date on the latest forms of treatment

2. Observing how the patient responds to treatment

3. Using alternative treatments if necessary

4. Discussing the patient's concerns freely and openly

5. Watching for complications that may arise

The patient should:

1. Keep scheduled appointments

2. Follow the agreed-upon treatment plan

3. Notify the office immediately about any complications or concerns

Treatments have the best chance for success when doctors and patients work together. If either party is not willing to do this, effective therapy will not result, and both the patient and the doctor will be frustrated and unhappy. Adhering to the suggested guidelines will result in a happier patient and better results.

CHAPTER 3

Spider Veins

WHAT ARE SPIDER VEINS?

Spider veins, or telangiectasias, are dilated bluish-red web-like veins that commonly develop on one or both legs. They can appear in clusters or as isolated threads. (Figure 1) A larger underlying vein, usually not readily visible, can sometimes contribute to the development of spider veins. In these cases, clearing an area of spider veins may also require treating the larger vein.

Spider veins are generally 0.1 to 1 mm in diameter, about the size of the tip of a pencil. Spider veins have no real function for your legs. They are just dilated, prominent skin veins. You have millions of other skin veins you can't see.

The presence of spider veins is generally regarded as a cosmetic condition. Ugly or unattractive visual appearance is a common complaint of patients with telangiectasias. Many people also report pain, itching, and burning, especially when the spider veins are in big clusters on the outside of the calf. Many medical conditions, either inherited, acquired, or the result of other treatments, can be associated with telangiectasias, but for most patients the unwelcome appearance is the main motivation for treatment.

WHY TREAT SPIDER VEINS?

Most people treat spider veins because of their unsightly appearance. A recent study showed that American women are more concerned

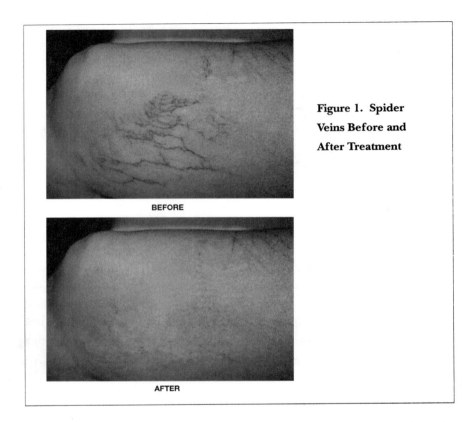

Figure 1. Spider
Veins Before and
After Treatment

BEFORE

AFTER

with lower extremity spider veins than almost any other cosmetic problem.[1] This problem seems to correlate with advancing age.[2] The incidence of leg telangiectasia in babies is less than 4%, whereas up to 35%
of adult American women and 10% of men have spider veins on the
legs.[3,4] Family history also seems to play a role. Studies have demonstrated up to a 90% positive family history in patients with spider leg
veins.[4] Most patients, however, develop spider veins during pregnancy,
and the veins become most severe after the third pregnancy. Only less
than one third of the patients developed spider veins before pregnancy,
and many of those were taking oral contraceptives at the time. Studies
conclude that the development of spider leg veins is probably partially
dependent on whether you are male or female. This problem may skip
generations and may have various levels of severity.[4,5] Many people treat
spider veins simply because they hurt.

RELATED CONDITIONS

Many other conditions are connected with spider vein formation. These include conditions such as port-wine stains, varicose veins, hormonal manipulations, injuries, infections, and radiation therapy skin changes.[6]

Port-wine stains affect up to 1% of the population.[7] Women are affected twice as often as men.[8] Although it is usually a sporadic event, there is a 10% familial incidence.[8] These lesions can occur on any part of the body, but most commonly occur on the face. Some can form open sores and bleed from minor trauma. Although they may be linked with other vascular diseases, they are often isolated findings.[6] Other blood vessel malformations, such as strawberry, capillary, and cavernous hemangiomas, can frequently be treated like spider veins. Examination under the microscope shows these lesions to be a variation of spider veins. Treatment should be performed only after a medical evaluation to insure that they are not part of a larger disease process.

Varicose veins can be associated with spider veins, and this can affect treatment. The proposed cause for this connection is the increased pressure in the venous system. As a result, blood flow reverses from the larger veins back toward the smaller veins including the veins near the skin, causing an opening and dilation of normally closed blood vessels.[9] In this case the treatment of spider veins may be best accomplished by treating the underlying varicose veins.

Hormonal factors such as pregnancy, estrogen therapy, and the use of steroid creams have also been linked to the development of spider veins.[6] It has been suggested that almost 70% of women develop spider veins during pregnancy,[9] although many of these disappear within 3 to 6 weeks after delivery. It has also been shown that pregnant women as well as those taking birth control pills can stretch their vein walls.[10] This increased distension has also been seen during the normal menstrual cycle. Not completely correlated with one specific hormone, this stretching seems to be related to both estrogen and progesterone levels, or may depend on the ratio of the two hormones.[6] This may explain why some women develop painful, dull-aching spider veins during their menstrual cycle.

Investigators have shown that excess estrogen may stimulate vein development or increase their ability to stretch.[11] This finding can be further supported in men who suffer with liver cirrhosis from alcohol. In these patients very high circulating estrogen levels are present, and spider veins are found all over their body.

High potency topical steroid skin preparations also cause the development of telangiectatic blood vessels.[8] Due to a change in the blood vessel wall, the blood vessels expand and become visible. Patients can sometimes see blood vessel dilation within 2 weeks of treatment with high-dose steroid creams.[6]

Injuries can lead to the development of new vessel growth. It is thought that these telangiectasias are the result of damage to existing blood vessels, which causes the release of factors that lead to new and increased blood vessel formation.

It has been shown that patients develop spider vein clusters after the fading of large bruises. Surgical incisions and skin cuts can also be associated with spider veins. Apparently, spider veins are the result of dilated and extended existing blood vessels. Some patients unfortunately develop quite an exaggerated spider vein response surrounding their scars,[6] possibly leading to a very bad cosmetic result.

Various infections have also caused spider veins; unfortunately, the exact mechanism is not clear. It has been shown that treatment of the underlying infection may occasionally resolve the spider vein formations.[6]

Radiation therapy for the treatment for various cancers is associated with the development of telangiectasias on the skin. At least 5% of the patients undergoing radiation therapy develop spider veins in the treatment field.[13] Apparently, blood vessels in the way of the beam are scarred, causing the remaining blood vessels that have not been as badly affected to dilate and become more visible to the eye.[14]

SUMMARY OF CAUSES

Spider veins are an extremely common disorder. They occur in up to one third of the adult population at any one time, with a high incidence in women. A variety of conditions have been associated with their

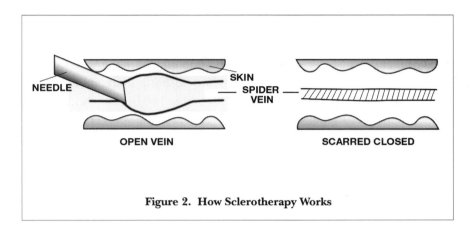

Figure 2. How Sclerotherapy Works

development; however their exact cause is still not known. It appears that the highest risk groups are those with a positive family history, females, and females who have been pregnant. Women placed on hormonal replacement therapy also appear to increase their risk for the development of spider veins.

TREATMENT OF SPIDER VEINS

The methods used to treat spider veins have only recently changed significantly. The advent of lasers and laser-like pulsed-light therapy has significantly altered the approach to treating vein problems, and may eventually replace the classic approach of sclerotherapy.

INJECTION SCLEROTHERAPY

Sclerotherapy, the use of needles to inject irritating medicine into a blood vessel, causing it to clot and subsequently scar closed, has been the mainstay of treatment for more than fifty years. (Figure 2) Better medicines have led to better results with decreased side effects to the areas around the veins, but the procedure can be quite tedious and time-consuming. The likelihood that the veins will come back rises as the diameter of the injected blood vessels increases. Even though the veins may come back, many patients seek this type of treatment. Until just recently, this was the only solution available.

Excellent results can be obtained using the "needle" technique, and studies have demonstrated a high degree of patient satisfaction. Cosmetic improvement has been demonstrated in up to 90% of the patients.[4]

Most patients require 4 to 6 sessions to have their spider veins treated. At The Vein Center in Memphis, 100 to 150 injections are often made with a very tiny needle during each session. Following sclerotherapy, patients should wear medical elastic compression stockings,[15] not over-the-counter support stockings.

Compression stockings must have a certain amount of "snugness" to be effective. "Support" hosiery have minimal leg "squeeze" and little medical benefit. Therefore, they are not recommended. Most physicians place patients in at least 20 to 30 mm Hg below-knee elastic compression stockings after below-knee injections are administered. If there are injections in the thighs as well, thigh-high or panty hose stockings are suggested.

The compression stockings' "squeeze" decreases from the ankle upward to insure appropriate drainage of the veins in the leg.[15] In most studies, an injected leg not supported with compression stockings has a higher chance of developing spider veins again. Patients should wear the compression stockings for 2 to 3 days around the clock after each treatment.[16]

For the first several days following the injections, the needle-stick sites are reinforced with cotton balls to increase the pressure. After 3 days, patients may take showers and remove their cotton balls and compression stockings. Some physicians believe patients should continue wearing the support stockings during the day for the next 2 weeks. Others say 6 weeks. Unfortunately, the optimum length of time for long-term compression in spider vein patients treated with sclerotherapy has not been established. At our vein center we believe the results are just as good with only 3 days of compression as with longer periods.

Complications related to sclerotherapy can be minimized when an experienced and dedicated physician does the treatment. Some patients experience a mild burning sensation while the sclerosing agent is entering the vein; however most patients are pleasantly surprised at the minimal discomfort during the treatment. Following treatment, some people experience bruising that generally fades over the next 3 to 4 weeks. Other complications that can occur are recurrence, hyperpigmentation, flare or cluster formation, ulceration, and very very rarely, superficial phlebitis or deep vein thrombosis.[17]

Although not a true complication of sclerotherapy, recurrence of spider veins is generally viewed as a problem by patients. This most commonly occurs when compression has not been adequately applied to the area of the spider vein sclerotherapy.[15] The larger the diameter of the vein treated by the injection technique, the more difficult it is to achieve a completely successful result. Because a larger volume of clotting or scarring material needs to be injected into a larger vessel, there is a greater likelihood of incomplete clotting. Subsequently, the vein can reopen in areas where scars were not fully formed.

Other things that increase the risk of recurrence include obesity, the use of estrogen-containing hormones, pregnancy, and a family history of spider veins. Excessive inflammation after the sclerotherapy injection may also play a role.[17]

Brown spots, which are due to an increase in pigmentation, occur in approximately 3 to 5% of patients following treatment. In most people they disappear in a few months, but they may last for up to a year. Very rarely they last longer than 5 years.[4] Although there is no good explanation for their cause, one reasonable theory suggests that a vein ruptures as the sclerosing solution is injected, then the solution and some blood leaks into the surrounding tissues and causes the spots.

In some patients a new cluster of very dense spider veins, known as a flare, may form in the area surrounding the vein just injected. This can look worse than the original problem. Flares can be treated with repeat sclerotherapy or other techniques discussed later in this chapter.

In less than 1% of patients, a small sore can occur at the injection site. This is called an ulcer. It is generally the size of a pencil eraser and will usually heal in several months with a small white scar. Usually it is caused because the scarring solution irritates the skin surrounding the spider vein. But with the development of new sclerosing solutions, this has become an uncommon problem.

Phlebitis and clots rarely occur in veins adjacent to spider veins. Clots can occur if sclerosing solution leaks into the surrounding larger veins, irritating them. In very rare instances, solution leaks into the deep vein system leading to clots similar to other deep vein thromboses. These would be treated like any other deep vein blood clots. Fortunately, this is a very rare occurrence when treating spider veins.[17] In our personal experience, we have never seen superficial or deep vein blood clots occur with this procedure.

LASERS AND PULSED-LIGHT TREATMENTS

In recent years, lasers have been used to treat spider veins. Laser is an acronym for *light amplification by stimulated emission of radiation*. A laser uses excited molecules to emit a specific wavelength of light in a very narrow beam. Many of the lasers now in use are visible spectrum instruments. Lasers for spider veins are very safe and are not associated with long-term side effects. The wavelength selected determines how deep the tissue penetration will be. Since these lasers use wavelengths longer than those used in x-rays or cobalt radiation therapy, they do not have the same concerns.

Because lasers are state of the art, a high level of patient acceptance has rapidly developed. Treatment without needles has led to increased patient demand. In addition, the reduction in needle puncture exposure has decreased contamination concerns for health care professionals, which has led to widespread acceptance in the medical community. Lastly, the publicity surrounding this "Star Wars" technology has led to meteoric dissemination of information through the news media. Some enthusiasm is justified, but some is excessive.

The lasers developed to treat spider veins work by producing a burst of high energy light that passes harmlessly through the skin and is selectively absorbed by the blood vessel. This should cause the blood vessel to heat up, destroying it by clotting, but without causing significant injury to the skin. (Figure 3) Although many lasers have been developed that were supposed to fulfill this promise, only a few

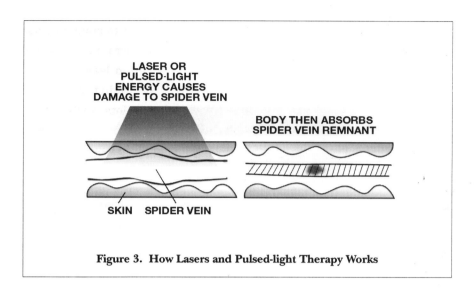

Figure 3. How Lasers and Pulsed-light Therapy Works

good lasers seem to dominate in spider vein treatment at this time. These produce very good spider vein destruction with minimal skin pigment changes and essentially no flare formation or scarring. They are only effective on small diameter spider veins, however, and can have variable success rates. Also, laser therapy can be mildly painful for the patient.[18,19]

In order to compensate for some of the heat discomfort patients feel on their skin, companies have developed skin-cooling devices in an effort to decrease the warm sensation without decreasing the energy delivered to the underlying targeted veins. Theoretically, this should allow patients to receive higher power exposure during each treatment and decrease the number of sessions required.[20,21] Several treatment sessions, though, are generally needed to eradicate spider veins with the lasers.

An occasional side effect of lasers is a form of bruising known as purpura, which is caused when heat ruptures the very tiny vessels that surround spider veins. Although not harmful, this may lengthen the time between treatments since most doctors won't treat an area again until purpura has resolved.[18]

Recently, an innovative laser-like pulsed-light source has been developed. This device causes the red blood cells to absorb heat directly. As a result, the vessel wall is slowly heated, which ultimately causes its destruction. Since this technology does not cause blood vessel rupture, there is little risk of post-treatment pigmentation changes and purpura. This technology apparently allows the entire vessel to clot without damaging the surrounding tissues or overlying skin. Furthermore, it allows the treatment of larger and more deeply situated leg veins than other laser technologies.[18,19]

The pulsed-light technique delivers its energy through a large crystal. This allows the rapid treatment of large areas with veins. To prevent nonspecific damage to the overlying skin, a cold clear gel is applied between the crystal light guide and the outer layer of the skin. The gel absorbs heat that may be reflected off the skin, preventing mild sunburn formation. Several treatment sessions are required to obtain the best results. Like the other lasers, it is mildly painful and feels like a snap of a rubber band on the skin or like a quick grease splatter when cooking.

Although all the lasers can effectively treat spider veins, our primary experience is with pulsed-light technology. The manufacturer of these instruments reports that blood vessels up to 3 mm in diameter can be effectively treated;[22] however, we have not used this method to treat vessels that large. It is our opinion that sclerotherapy is better for larger spider veins. On the other hand, pulsed-light has given extremely good results in the treatment of typical small spider veins. Patients have reported minimal discomfort, the treatment sessions are well-tolerated, and patients have been quite happy with the results. Minimal side effects have been noted. Furthermore, any treatment that does not require compression hose is greatly appreciated by patients, especially during the summer and in warm climates.

Recently, an extension of pulsed-light therapy was developed for treating deeper and larger vessels that did not get good results when laser treated and therefore required injection sclerotherapy.[23] Investigators have reported a 93% success rate in vessel closure, with 80%

requiring only one treatment. Side effects were minimal.[23] Although we have no personal experience with this system as yet, a well-respected vein care physician has confirmed these early findings in patients he has treated.[24]

Lasers and laser-like therapies may have some advantages over traditional injection sclerotherapy for treating spider veins. The lasers rapidly heat and clot the blood vessels, so leakage of blood cells into the surrounding tissue, thought to lead to temporary or permanent pigment changes, is decreased. Furthermore, the rare sores caused when scarring solution leaked into the tissue surrounding the vein are avoided. Also, flare formation has not been commonly associated with laser treatments. Finally, unusual allergic reactions to the sclerosing solution by individual patients cannot occur when a laser is used.

SUMMARY OF TREATMENTS

Injection sclerotherapy has been the mainstay of spider vein treatment for the last fifty years. As the scarring solutions have improved, so have the results. Complication rates have decreased to very acceptable levels, and the only problems that commonly persist are the recurrence of veins and the occasional development of very dense vein clusters known as flares.

As technology has expanded, it has penetrated into the area of spider vein treatment. The use of lasers and laser-like therapies for spider veins has been met with widespread enthusiasm both from patients and doctors. The ability to avoid needles and their associated health risks means these machines are here to stay. Also, eliminating pigmentation changes and flare formation is nice from a cosmetic standpoint.

Both treatment methods work very well for spider veins. The approach used will depend on the doctors involved, patient preference, and the clinical situation. We often mix and match the two techniques in the same patient to get the best results.

WHAT PEOPLE LIKE YOU HAVE TO SAY

"When I was young, I had pretty legs. Not the kind you dream about, just attractive legs. Now after three children my legs look like road maps. I have a major avenue on my legs named after each child. I hate to wear shorts and I won't wear a bathing suit. What can I do?"

Kathy M., age 43, a former aerobics instructor, now a homemaker

Problem: Diffuse spider veins on both legs.

The Doctor's Recommendations: Treatment with pulsed-light laser-like therapy, with the sessions spaced 3 to 4 weeks apart.

Results: Nice clearance of almost all the spider veins over the 4-month treatment period. Four sessions were required.

Total cost: $1,100 (4 sessions at $275 per session).

The Patient's Comments Post-Treatment: "This was a piece of cake. For years I've been avoiding treatment since I didn't want needle sticks and I didn't want to wear those heavy stockings. But with the laser there was nothing to it! At first I didn't think it was working, but over the next couple of weeks the veins just started disappearing. In less than two hours of total treatment I was finally rid of those nasty spider veins. Now for the first time since I was in my twenties I can wear a bathing suit when I take my kids to the pool. I won't be so embarrassed when I go back to work and start changing in the locker room again. I did get one spot that looked a little sunburned for a few weeks, but it didn't hurt. Compared to those big blue patches, I'll take a small red one for a week anytime."

What about the cost?: "I wish insurance would cover this. It's like any other medical expense as far as I'm concerned. It makes me feel good about myself, and I'm no longer afraid to go out in shorts. If they pay for other therapies to get over fears and make someone feel better about themselves, then why won't they pay for this? I think $1,100 was a small price to pay for all the things I plan on doing this summer in shorts and a bathing suit."

*

"I'm 59 years old and I've been a widow for the last seven years. I never cared much about my spider veins. But now I've met the most wonderful man. He wants us to get married in eight weeks. We're going on our honeymoon to the Caribbean and I want to look nice in a bathing suit. I want the fastest possible way to get rid of these nasty spider veins."

Mary S., age 59, a retail sales clerk and mother of two grown children

Problem: Diffuse spider veins on both legs with the desire for a very rapid resolution.

The Doctor's Recommendations: Treatment with injection sclerotherapy on a weekly treatment schedule.

Results: Good clearance of virtually all the spider veins after 5 treatment sessions. We probably could have cleared everything in 6 sessions, but we wanted to allow 2 weeks for the mild bruising from the needle sticks to clear prior to the wedding and honeymoon.

Total cost: $1,485 (5 sclerotherapy sessions at $275.00 per session and a one-time charge of $120 for the panty-hose-length compression stockings that she wore throughout the treatment course.

The Patient's Comments Post-Treatment: "I wish I would have done this years ago. Once I got used to the little needle sticks, it was no big deal. I only had a little bit of the bruising that they warned me about. Once I got used to the heavy support stockings, they actually felt pretty good on my legs. I am glad though that it was winter, since I think they would be hot in the summer."

What about the cost?: "Well, you always want it to be cheaper, but most of all I wanted it to work! I'm starting a new life and I want to feel good about myself. I don't want my new husband to think I have ugly legs. It took me 30 years to get like this. Fifteen hundred divided by 30 is $50.00 per year. I think that's a pretty small price to pay to make me look better. That's less than I spend each year on lipstick alone."

CHAPTER 4
Varicose Veins

WHAT ARE VARICOSE VEINS?

The World Health Organization defines varicose veins as "saccular dilatation of the veins which are often tortuous."[1] The term "varicose" is derived from the Greek word for "grape-like." These abnormally shaped veins have valves that don't work properly. When a valve malfunctions, pressure can build inside the vein, resulting in the abnormal shape. (Figure 1)

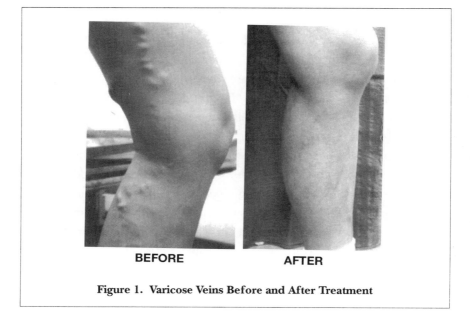

BEFORE   AFTER

Figure 1. Varicose Veins Before and After Treatment

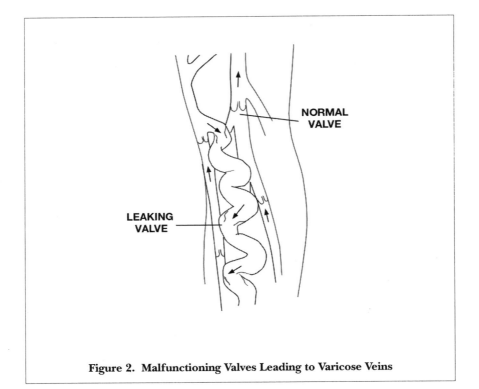

Figure 2. Malfunctioning Valves Leading to Varicose Veins

Vein valves are the weakest point in the vessel; they appear to be the weak link that leads to the development of varicose veins. When valves leak, blood pools in a vein rather than emptying out of it, and turbulent blood flow occurs. The vein then dilates. The more it enlarges, the more this affects other valves down the line. (Figure 2) The main theory explaining why varicose veins develop proposes that weak vein walls stretch when exposed to high pressure. As these walls stretch, the veins shape changes, causing the valves to work improperly.[2] Whichever came first, the abnormal valves or the weak walls, the end result is the same—abnormally functioning blood vessels that can cause a variety of symptoms. One American health survey found that nearly 50% of the patients with varicose veins had occasional symptoms, but 18% admitted to discomfort, from frequent to continuous.[3] A large number of causes have been blamed for the development of varicose veins. The most popular ones include heredity, gender, weight, and hormone therapy.[2,4]

WHAT CAUSES VARICOSE VEINS?

It is known that varicose veins run in families. Studies have shown that up to 85% of children evidence varicose veins when both parents are affected.[5] A study on identical twins found that 75% of the time both were affected, whereas same-sex fraternal twins had only about a 50% incidence of varicose veins.[6]

It does not appear however, that people develop varicose veins just because they have a positive family history.[7] There seems to be multiple other factors, which may include their job and hormonal influences. Although it is clear that varicose vein problems run in families, the absolute cause is not yet known.

Gender clearly plays a role in the development of varicose veins. More than one half of adult men and two thirds of adult women have physically identifiable varicosities.[8] The cause for the percentage difference may be hormones and pregnancy.[4,9] These two effects may be one and the same though, since many pregnancy changes are hormonally regulated. The other peak time for developing varicose veins in women appears to be at menopause, another time when hormonal changes occur.

It is unclear which of the two female hormones, estrogen or progesterone, plays the main role in the development of varicose veins.[4,9] Some feel it is the ratio of these two hormones that is most important. Hormonal levels change most dramatically during pregnancy and menopause, and these changes can be further compounded by birth control pills throughout a woman's life, and by hormone replacement therapy after menopause.

Estrogen and progesterone are produced by the ovaries and the adrenal glands in women. The level of these hormones rises and falls cyclically. Prior to the onset of menstruation, progesterone levels rise. With the onset of bleeding, progesterone falls and estrogen rises. Estrogen levels are highest at mid cycle when the ovaries release eggs. Researchers have found that about 25% of women with varicose veins have premenstrual pain in their varices.[10] Progesterone levels rise dramatically during the first several weeks of pregnancy. After that, estrogen levels rise and stay above normal until the completion of pregnancy. As menopause approaches, estrogen and progesterone levels elevate and fall radically. This may cause the host of symptoms that perimenopausal women describe. Furthermore, the many signs of premenstrual syndrome (PMS) may also be linked to the rise and fall of various hormones.

Estrogen and progesterone can affect veins in many ways. Some researchers believe that estrogen or progesterone or both allow for the stretching of vein walls. Some researchers have found a 20 to 30% increase in vein diameter during the menstrual cycle, with up to a 150% increase during pregnancy. Estrogen and progesterone may cause smooth muscle relaxation that softens the walls of the veins, which in turn makes it more difficult for the vein valves to close.[4,9]

Leg veins are under greater pressure during pregnancy because the womb blocks some of the blood return to the heart. Pregnancy also increases the amount of blood circulating in the body. As blood volume increases up to 150% above normal, congestion leads to increases in vein pressure and may play a direct role in the development of varicose veins.

After delivery, many women may find that their varicose veins and their symptoms go away. Again, this is thought to be related to changes in hormone levels. Many physicians recommend waiting 6 to 12 weeks following delivery of your baby to determine how many varicose veins will be left.[9]

Obesity and excess weight have long been associated with the development of varicose veins.[4,11-13] The exact mechanism is not completely understood, but it is believed that increased weight leads to increased pressure on the veins. This is similar to the increased pressure on the pelvic veins from the enlarging baby during pregnancy, or the increased intra-abdominal pressure in patients with chronic constipation.[14] It is thought that the increased pressure in the pelvic veins is transmitted down to the leg veins, eventually causing injury to the leg vein valves. Some studies, however, have shown that when the patient's age is correlated to obesity, no significant association is found.[15,16] The presence of the varicose veins may be solely the result of advancing age.[4] In one area, however, obesity seems to play a significant role in varicose veins in women: when varicose veins occur with the skin changes of venous stasis.[12,13] This problem will be further described in the chapter entitled Chronic Venous Insufficiency.

Crossing your legs has been commonly thought to lead to varicose veins, possibly because the blood attempting to return from the legs to the heart is blocked. Leg crossing is thought to cause outside pressure on the vein; however this has never been scientifically verified. However, prolonged standing including jobs with lots of standing have been shown to correlate with an increased incidence of varicose veins.[17]

Prolonged sitting in a chair may also be a cause for concern.[18,19] Sitting may produce some external compression on the back of the thigh, which may cause a resistance to blood return. This has significant implications for people who travel for long periods of time. Leg vein blood clots and blood clots that go to the lungs have occurred in many people after prolonged travel in the sitting position. Despite the fact that many of these people may have had preexisting vein problems, extensive chair sitting just seems to add another dimension.

COMMON PROBLEMS ASSOCIATED WITH VARICOSE VEINS: PHLEBITIS AND THROMBOPHLEBITIS

Phlebitis, an inflamed vein wall, is the most common problem associated with varicose veins. It usually develops in a branch of the superficial saphenous system. Most people with varicose veins will have at least one attack of phlebitis during their lifetime.[20]

A dull ache is usually the first sign of phlebitis, often accompanied by slight swelling and tenderness over the course of the involved vein. Next the area becomes pink, warm, and tender. As the process continues, the skin overlying the vein becomes red hot to the touch, and the leg hurts, especially when moved or squeezed.[20]

The treatment for phlebitis is generally conservative. Patients are encouraged to walk, even though initially this is uncomfortable. They should also wear elastic compression stockings. Aspirin is frequently prescribed for both its anti-inflammatory and mild blood-thinning effects. With time, the inflammation will resolve, the redness goes away, and the overlying skin can develop a brown discoloration, either temporary or permanent.

When phlebitis occurs alone, it is usually not serious. When the inflamed saphenous vein goes on to develop a clot, it is called thrombophlebitis, and this is a matter of serious concern. In the absence of cancer, thrombophlebitis of the leg is almost always associated with varicose veins.[21,22] It has been estimated that up to 50% of those with varicose veins will suffer with superficial thrombophlebitis at least once in their lives.[23] This problem increases in frequency with advancing age, inactivity, and prolonged bed rest.[24] Each year 123,000 people in the United States are expected to suffer with this condition.[25]

Superficial thrombophlebitis can occur after injury to the varicose veins or with slow or blocked blood flow in the veins.[26] Fifty percent of the cases are spontaneous and without an obvious cause.[21]

The symptoms of thrombophlebitis are similar to those of isolated phlebitis. A dull aching sensation and mild swelling are usually present. Warmth overlying the involved skin is also common. With time, however, you can feel a hard, cord-like structure along the involved vein. The treatment for this will be given in more detail under the section on blood clots. Due to the significant discomfort, most patients rapidly seek treatment, which allows more significant problems to be avoided.

SUMMARY

No one knows exactly why varicose veins develop. Varicose veins are more a group of problems than an isolated finding. Frequently, they are associated with heredity, age, and lifestyle. Varicose veins have dilated walls and valves that no longer work properly, which allows blood to pool in these veins. Whether the chicken (stretched vein walls) or the egg (leaky valves) comes first has not been clearly determined, but we can say that this is a very common problem affecting millions of people in the United States. Abnormal vein valves play a major role in many of the problems that will later be discussed.

TREATMENT OF VARICOSE VEINS

The treatment of varicose veins varies widely throughout the world. Volumes of medical textbooks have been written addressing the most common treatment techniques. This chapter will touch on the main modalities for treatment: compression therapy, injection sclerotherapy, and surgical removal.

ELASTIC COMPRESSION STOCKINGS

Damage caused to vein walls by abnormally functioning valves and the resulting pooled blood is not reversible, but measures have been developed to prevent the progression of the problem. Compression stockings, touched on in the chapter about spider veins, are believed to work by externally supporting bulging vein walls that lie under the skin. As these veins are compressed, more strength is given to their walls than when stockings are not worn. This prevents the pooling of the blood within these vessels. Stockings also help to control leg swelling, probably by forcing the edema fluid back into the veins as the tissues under the skin are squeezed.[27,28] It is thought that compression reconfigures the leaky vein valves and restores their functional effectiveness.

Since venous diseases tend to show progression, a consistent compression therapy treatment program is required. The fit of the stockings is extremely important. Since elastic stretches, the stockings should be replaced every 4 to 6 months. Over-the-counter, off-the-shelf stockings labelled as beneficial for whatever ails one's legs are probably not as effective due to inadequate levels of compression. They are not a good substitute for high quality, properly fitted, elastic compression stockings.

Another purpose for medical compression hosiery is to maintain the results of other treatments and to avoid subsequent complications. They appear to decrease pain in affected legs and prevent relapses of symptoms such as swelling and phlebitis.

In some countries, the long-term problems of varicose veins and other vein problems are felt to be so significant that compression stockings are issued by the government as a preventative and therapeutic modality. In Germany, two pairs of compression stockings have been allowed each year with the permission of their national health insurance program.[28] In our country, this approach is not as readily accepted. As a preventive device alone, compression stockings are generally not covered by health insurance policies. As a therapeutic device following the development of complications, compression stockings may sometimes be covered. For example, the occasional insurance company will reimburse compression treatment for varicose veins with inflammation, varicose veins with open sores, varicose veins with both sores and inflammation, or varicose veins that have been bleeding. Thus, patients are often only being allowed reimbursed treatment for prescription stockings after complications of the varicose veins have occurred. This is far more costly, risky, and uncomfortable for the patient. Also many of the problems may have been avoidable had there been proper early attention.

By themselves, compression stockings are generally not a good long-term treatment alternative for varicose veins, falling short of other treatment modalities due to compliance problems when patients must wear these stocking for many years, and also because the damaged or abnormal vein has not been treated. An exception to this may be the most elderly or sickest patients where the physicians are attempting to simply treat symptoms and avoid more taxing procedures. Compression stockings should be viewed as an essential part of a larger treatment plan in patients with varicose veins.

SCLEROTHERAPY

For the past sixty years, primary sclerotherapy has been used by many clinicians to treat varicose veins. The technique of injecting solutions to scar a vein closed is the same as for spider veins. The specific places in the superficial vein system that control vein filling when the patient goes from lying to standing must be diagnosed and then injected with solution.[29] Multiple books and papers have been written on the best ways to do this.[29-33]

Excellent initial results have been described from many centers. Some report up to 85% relief of symptoms.[34] To improve long-term results, others have added the limited surgical procedure of tying off the leaking vein valve in the groin. Following recovery, sclerotherapy of the varicose veins is performed.[35]

Much of the original thrust toward sclerosing symptomatic varicose veins was for people in whom surgery was contraindicated.[36] Next, it was used to treat recurrent or missed veins after surgery. Finally, it was touted as a less costly and less uncomfortable procedure than the classical varicose vein stripping operation.[37,38] From these starting points, others have enhanced the technique so it can be used on anyone with varicose veins.

Unfortunately the long-term results of injection sclerotherapy for big varicose veins (greater than a .25 of an inch in diameter) have been poor. Failure rates as high as 88 to 100% have been recorded.[37,39] The biggest problem with injection sclerotherapy for varicose veins seems to be that its benefits are short-lived. Multiple studies published in the medical literature have shown that within 3 to 4 years there is at least a 60 to 80% recurrence rate for varicose veins that should have been surgically removed, but were instead treated with sclerotherapy alone or in conjunction with compression stockings.[40-43]

Multiple sessions, such as those used to treat spider veins, are required until all of the varicosities have adequately been injected. In contrast, surgery can take care of virtually all the varicosities in one session. Complications similar to those encountered with sclerotherapy treatment of spider veins are seen with this treatment for varicose veins.

Recently there has been growing enthusiasm for the use of ultrasound guided sclerotherapy, which uses sound waves to completely visualize the vein under the skin. It was developed to make sure that the varicose vein was adequately treated, hopefully decreasing the recurrence rate.[44-46] Some have voiced concern that long-term studies will again show a high recurrence rate.[47] Others, however, have embraced the technique.[48-50] Early studies suggest good results, but long-term data are still needed prior to widespread acceptance of this treatment.

Several "experts" have been very critical of sclerotherapy for varicose veins,[51,52] but it clearly has a role in treating varicose veins, and the techniques are here to stay. It is our opinion, as well as that of a well-respected committee of vein care specialists,[53] that small varicose veins, usually those less than about 3 mm in size (about .25 in. in diameter), can effectively be treated with sclerotherapy.

Due to the high reported recurrence rates following sclerotherapy, large varicose veins require surgical removal to get the best results. The combination of varicose vein surgery with sclerotherapy may be the best management approach in many patients. The proper role of sclerotherapy in the treatment of varicose veins appears to be after larger varicosities have been surgically removed. Small residual varicosities can then be effectively treated with sclerotherapy. This plan seems to lend itself to good results with the least chance the varicose veins will return.

SURGERY

Over the years, operations for varicose veins have evolved from a very painful procedure to the present day outpatient minimally invasive technique. Hippocrates gets the first credit for varicose vein treatment in 370 B.C., recommending multiple punctures to remove the veins.[54] In A.D. 200, Galen used a hook to pull out the veins.[55] In A.D. 400, the Egyptians described modern therapy for varicose veins: "cut skin, expose varix, insert probe under it...pull out varix and cut."[56] Aegineta in A.D. 650 suggested ligation, division, and compression therapy.[57] But it was not until the 1950s that monumental contributions in vein surgery evolved.[57]

Since the thought of surgery scares most people, a basic discussion of the pro's and con's is needed. The concept is quite straightforward: remove the bad veins, thereby forcing the blood back to the heart through healthy veins with working valves. From this one simple idea, vein surgery has evolved.

Surgery can be chosen over injection sclerotherapy for several reasons. The most important seems to be better treatment of larger veins.[58] Other indications include recurrent episodes of thrombophlebitis, bleeding from the varicose veins, and the skin changes of chronic venous insufficiency that will be discussed in a later chapter.[59] It can even be performed after there has been a blood clot in the deep veins of the leg, but the utmost care and a perfect technique are required.[60]

When surgery has been chosen, physicians should strive to achieve three main goals:

1. Permanent removal of all the varicose veins
2. Excellent cosmetic results
3. A minimum number of complications[58]

Prior to the 1980s, surgeons made multiple incisions overlying every visible lump and bump of the varicosities to remove the diseased veins. Although this was an effective treatment, multiple incisions and scars were present, often leading to a long recovery and a poor cosmetic result.

Another technique commonly used, even in the current era, is the classic vein stripping. This technique usually requires either general or spinal anesthesia and frequently a trip to a hospital or surgery center. First, an incision is made in the groin, usually hidden in the bikini line, and another incision is made inside of the ankle. Then, a long instrument is inserted into the vein that starts at the ankle and ends in the groin. The vein is then tied to this "stripper." As the instrument is pulled out, the vein comes with it. By removing the entire saphenous vein in this fashion, there is a permanent change of blood flow in the superficial system, forcing the superficial blood to travel back to the heart through the deep veins. This technique removes the entire saphenous vein from the ankle to the groin. Unfortunately, it also causes injury to the tissues surrounding the vein and leaves a large tunnel in which blood can accumulate. This procedure has been associated with considerable pain and discomfort, and a prolonged recovery is also often required. Although still commonly performed, this technique leaves something to be desired as far as pain, injury, expense, and recovery time. This procedure has given varicose vein surgery a bad name.

Present day state-of-the-art surgical procedures for varicose veins, practiced by many surgeons around the country, are now based on techniques used in other forms of surgery. In the 1990s the development of minimally invasive varicose vein surgery completely revolutionized the treatment of this disorder.[61] Through the use of special instruments, this disorder can be surgically treated through very small incisions with little to no pain. The development of tiny incision surgery for varicose veins, known as ambulatory phlebectomy, along with the removal of the veins under local or regional anesthesia, has eliminated hospitalizations. No longer are general or spinal anesthesia used, and rapid recovery is almost always seen. It has also led to a remarkable decrease in the cost of surgery. Furthermore, the cosmetic result is far superior. Since very small 1 to 3 mm incisions are used, almost no scars are present. This technique also makes it possible to remove only the abnormal areas, rather than stripping the entire vein from groin to ankle. The patient then keeps the normal portions of the greater saphenous vein, which can later be used for operations such as heart bypass surgery if needed.

Using very early instruments for this new operation, a 10-year recurrence rate of only 7% was reported in close to 2,000 operations.[62] Others have reported 0% recurrence at 1 and 2 years in over 1,000 procedures.[63] Complication rates have been minimal.[63,64] Excellent cosmetic results have been obtained using these methods at The Vein Center in Memphis as well as in others around the country.[63] This is our approach of choice for treating all varieties and combinations of large varicose veins.

With the described advances in surgical techniques, varicose vein surgery can now routinely be performed in a vein center or an outpatient surgery center. Previously, surgery required a full day or an overnight stay in a hospital, with associated charges for laboratory tests, supplies, the operating room, anesthesia, and the recovery room: amounting to approximately $8,000 to $10,000 or more depending on the area of the area of the country. The surgeon's fee could be between $2,500 and $3,500 for one leg, double that amount for two legs. Now, with the new techniques, significant cost savings to the patient and the insurance company are possible.

These new vein surgery procedures are all done in the operating room at our free-standing vein center. This saves the patient and the insurance company money. The methods that we have described, depending on the extent of surgery required, cost less than $2,500 for each procedure, including the surgeon's fee, local anesthetic, and all supplies. Furthermore, an entire day is not lost by the patient, who must arrive two hours prior to the procedure at a hospital or surgery center and then spend time postoperatively in a recovery room. Treatment in an office setting, along with a reduced cost of approximately one fourth the previous charge for varicose vein surgery, truly places this in the realm of a minimally invasive procedure. In addition, the use of local or nerve-block anesthesia eliminates the long period of recovery. Patients walk out of our office at the end of the procedure, and virtually all return to work or their normal household activities the next day.

More than half of our patients report that they don't take anything for pain once they leave our center. Furthermore, with the ability to return to work the next day, thousands of dollars in lost wages and productivity for both the patient and employer are eliminated. This savings alone far outweighs the entire cost of treating varicose veins at a vein center.

TREATMENT SUMMARY

Varicose vein treatment appears to be coming around full circle. In the early years surgery was the only option. But due to the painful operations used and the long recovery required, it was mainly used for the worst conditions. Sclerotherapy then became popular as an accepted treatment method, especially for doctors not trained in surgery and for patients who didn't want to "go under the knife." Unfortunately, the results of sclerotherapy for larger varicose veins, which are often the most symptomatic, did not stand the test of time. Recurrence rates as high as 100% were reported as early as 1 year after treatment. Although the risk of recurrence is high following injection sclerotherapy, many still prefer the possibility of the veins coming back to the thought of surgery. Heavy compression stockings were then used alone to rapidly treat the symptoms and prevent the veins from worsening. Although effective in making the patients' legs feel better, stockings didn't fix the main problem of the leaking valves and are now understood to play an essential part in complementing other forms of therapy. So now we're back to the surgical treatment of "large" varicose veins.

With the development of special operations for this problem, and by customizing the treatment plan and surgery for each individual patient, excellent long-term results are obtained. Using today's advanced instruments and performing the procedures under local anesthesia in free-standing vein centers, minimal discomfort and short recovery times are common. Also, costs have been significantly reduced by making this an office procedure comparable in expense or often even less expensive than sclerotherapy. As knowledge and training of physicians in this new approach continues, we hope that more of the millions of people troubled with varicose veins will seek earlier treatment. This action alone will save years of needless suffering and expensive complications.

WHAT PEOPLE LIKE YOU HAVE TO SAY

"For years I have had throbbing, pulling sensations in my legs that got better when I lay down at night. But as a nurse I work 8- to 10-hour shifts and stand almost all the time. I've tried support stockings and good shoes, but they just don't help. I used to feel some bumps in my legs, but since I lost some weight I can now really see the varicose veins. That's where I'm sore. Is there anything we can do? I have to keep working and I can't afford to lose much time from work. I'm a single mother with two school-age children."

Nancy K., age 36, a full-time mom and full-time nurse

Problem: Painful varicose vein from the ankle to just below the knee.

The Doctor's Recommendations: Surgical removal of the varicose vein in a vein center or an office setting under local anesthesia using state-of-the-art, minimally invasive microsurgical techniques.

Results: There was nice removal of the symptomatic varicose vein and its side branches in the calf. The patient was placed in below-knee elastic compression stockings for about two weeks postoperatively.

She had the procedure performed in the office on a Friday afternoon. She spent about 2 hours at the office. None of the incisions were large enough to require stitches. All of them could be closed with butterfly bandages, resulting in essentially no visible scar after 4 to 6 weeks. She was able to return to work at full duty on Monday, the third day after surgery, and could have returned sooner if needed. She spent the weekend doing her normal household and motherly activities, with the only restrictions being no high-impact aerobics or jogging for the first 3 days. Her total time lost from work was half a day, and it appeared to all others that it was a normal weekend for her.

Total cost: $2,410 (initial physician consultation, $100; venous ultrasound of the leg to localize the varicose vein and help determine the extent of surgery required, $325; surgeons' fee, $1,500; surgical supply charge, $425; below-knee compression stockings, $60). These charges should all be covered by health insurance, with the amount of payment varying by geographic location, policy type, and which health plans you and your physicians are members of. In our experience, most patients have had good cooperation from their insurance companies for this problem and end up paying about $500 out of pocket. This is far less than if surgery had been performed in a hospital with its attendant preoperative, laboratory, facility, operating room, recovery room, and anesthesiology charges, which combined with the surgeons fee of at least $1,500 are often well in excess of $10,000 to $15,000. With a 20% deductible that generally places out-of-pocket costs in the range of $2,000 to $3,000. That does not include the cost of time lost from work or the discomfort and personal recovery needed when older surgical methods are used.

The Patient's Comments Post-Treatment: "This was easy. Going to the dentist's office is much worse than this for me. I put the prescribed numbing cream on my skin before I left work to go to The Vein Center. By the time they started, I didn't even feel the needle sticks from the local anesthesia. I spent 2 hours at the office on a Friday afternoon and only had to use half a day of sick leave. The weekend was like any other in my household, except my kids volunteered to clean up more than usual. I would recommend this to anybody who needs this kind of surgery. The compression stockings that I wore immediately after the veins were removed made my legs feel so good that now I wear them all the time at work under my uniform pants."

*

"Years ago, after the birth of my second child, I had the varicose veins in my left leg stripped. It was horrible! I was in the hospital for 3 days and it took me weeks to fully recover. They had me in bulky bandages, and then I had to wear these ugly white support stockings for 6

months. When I started getting varicose veins in my right leg, I just ignored them for as long as possible. Now I can't put it off any longer. My leg aches all the time and my foot swells by the end of the day. I sure hope it's better than the last time."

Carol N., age 59, a retail sales clerk at a department store, wife, and mother of four grown children and grandmother of six

Problem: Symptomatic greater saphenous vein varicosities from groin to ankle.

The Doctor's Recommendations: Surgical removal of the varicose vein in a vein center or office setting under local anesthesia using state-of-the-art, minimally invasive microsurgical techniques. Due to the limitation on the amount of local anesthesia that can be safely given at one time, 2 procedures will have to be performed spaced at least 1 day apart. The thigh portion with a ligation of the vein in the groin will be done first, followed by removal of the vein from the ankle to the knee at the second surgery.

Results: Excellent removal of the varicose vein from ankle to groin during 2 surgeries staged 3 days apart. The patient was placed in panty hose elastic compression stockings for about 2 weeks postoperatively. The procedures were performed Friday afternoon and the following Monday morning at The Vein Center. She took the next 2 days off and 3 days later was able to return to her normal work routine standing and selling cosmetics as a retail clerk. The total time lost from work was 3.5 days. She could have gone to work the next day, but had some sick days to use or lose. On her first postoperative visit a small 2 mm branch varicosity was still present on the inside of her calf. This was injected with sclerosing solution, and she continued to wear her compression stockings for 2 more weeks, which she would have done anyway. On her final visit at 1 month, she had no residual varicosities.

She ended up with 4 skin stitches for the 2 surgeries. One was on her ankle and three were in the groin. Everything else was small enough to close with butterfly bandages, resulting in essentially invisible scars at 6 weeks.

Total cost: $4,395 (initial physician consultation, $100; venous ultrasound of the leg to localize the extent of surgery required, $325; surgeons' fee for first phase, $1,500; surgical supply charge, $425; panty hose compression stockings, $120; surgeons' fee for the second procedure $1,500; surgical supply charge for the second procedure, $425.) As with the previous case, these charges should all be covered by health insurance. The out-of-pocket expenses and realized savings should be similar as well.

The Patient's Comments Post-Treatment: "I was dreading this for years. But this was nothing like the last time. I started laughing when the doctor told me we could do this in the office under local anesthesia, that I would need only acetaminophen or ibuprofen for pain, and that I could be back at work in several days. Last time I wasn't able to work for a month. The incisions were so small I couldn't even see where they took the veins out. I wish I would have done this sooner. Anyone that does this the old way is crazy. Who cares if it took 2 sessions? There was no pain and I could do whatever I wanted after them."

CHAPTER 5

Unwanted Veins on Your Face

WHAT ARE FACIAL SPIDER VEINS?

Spider veins or telangiectasias are very common on the face, especially on the nose, mid-cheeks, and chin. Similar to those on the legs, they are often red in color with multiple branches. (Figure 1) Blue veins are far less common. They are usually found on the chin. Little cherry red hemangiomas, although not true spider veins, are often grouped and treated just like facial spider veins.

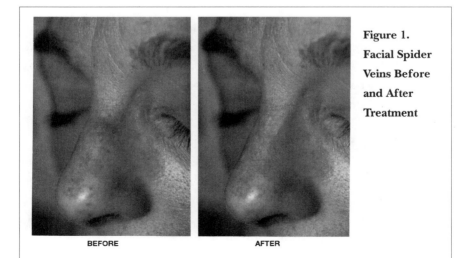

BEFORE

AFTER

Figure 1.
Facial Spider
Veins Before
and After
Treatment

Facial telangiectasia typically appear in preschool and school-age children. As many as 50% of children less than 15 years old have at least one spot.[1] In adults this number is approximately 15%. This means that most childhood facial veins do not need treatment. They will resolve on their own.

WHAT CAUSES FACIAL SPIDER VEINS?

Many of the causes of facial veins are similar to those of other spider veins. These include hormonal factors, and injuries such as cuts, surgical incisions, and rhinoplasties (nose jobs). Radiation therapy to the face and neck are also commonly associated with spider vein formation.[2] These veins can also be part of a variety of medical conditions including collagen vascular diseases such as lupus erythematosus. These conditions are beyond the scope of this book. Readers should ask their physicians about specific medical problems.

Facial spider veins are most commonly seen in those with fair skin complexions. They are probably the result of vessel wall weaknesses made worse by chronic sun exposure.[3] Medicines such as topical steroid creams can make the situation worse.[2]

COMMON TREATMENTS FOR
FACIAL SPIDER VEINS

Most people with facial veins present for treatment for cosmetic reasons, but some patients may develop bleeding from or into the skin.[3] Since most office visits are the result of concerns about personal appearance, treatment should aim to avoid unsightly scarring. The most common approaches include injection sclerotherapy, lasers, electrosurgery, and pulsed-light therapy.

The principals of facial sclerotherapy are similar to those for spider veins of the leg. Facial veins don't respond as well, however, and are prone to complications.[3] Great care should be taken to choose a physician who has significant experience with these problems because compression therapy cannot easily be performed on the face for any length of time. Hence, one of the prime components in the success of sclerotherapy (prolonged compression) is lacking. Results in general are less than excellent.

Frequently sclerotherapy must be combined with another treatment modality. We believe that other forms of therapy are usually safer and give a better cosmetic result. Facial sclerotherapy should be reserved for select circumstances under the guidance of an experienced clinician.

Electrosurgery, also known as electrodesiccation, is still commonly used to treat facial spider veins. A needle is placed into the vessel every 2 to 3 mm along its course. A very small electrical current is then passed through the needle, causing dehydration in the tissue immediately surrounding it. Destruction of the vein and a very limited area around the vein occurs.[3] Unfortunately, multiple treatments are usually required, but experienced physicians can produce excellent results. To minimize the risk of scarring, it is best reserved for very small facial veins.

A wide variety of lasers have been used to treat facial veins; therefore only a general review can be given. Several give excellent results with minimal risks.[3] Lasers cause vein destruction by vaporizing the water within the blood cells. A specific wavelength of light is chosen to obtain the desired depth of tissue penetration. The pulse duration should be chosen so that it is brief enough to cause the desired effect on the vein, but produces only minimal damage to the surrounding tissue. Patients usually obtain good to excellent results. A few patients will develop some bruising in the area treated,[3] but this usually resolves in 1 to 2 weeks. It is thought that this bruising, called purpura, results from heating the tiny microscopic veins surrounding the spider vein to a temperature higher than the boiling point of blood, causing the vein to "pop." Blood from this overheated vessel then oozes into the surrounding tissue causing the discoloration.[4] Although transient, this occasional problem can be temporarily disturbing since it is an additional blemish on the face.

Laser-like pulsed-light therapy has also been used to treat facial spider veins. As with leg telangiectasias, the pulsed-light causes the red blood cells to absorb heat, resulting in blood vessel clotting and vessel wall destruction. Since blood does not boil in the vessel, purpura can usually be prevented, as can the dark pigmentation spots that are thought to occur when a blood vessel ruptures and stains the surrounding tissue.

At our vein center, pulsed-light therapy has been very effective in rapidly and completely treating facial veins, usually in only a few sessions. In some instances 40 or 50 spots have been treated at a time. Patients generally experience some mild redness and minimal swelling in the region, which resolves in hours. Patient satisfaction has been quite high with this technique.

SUMMARY

Facial spider veins are a very common problem, especially for fair-skinned individuals. No one knows exactly why they develop, but a reasonable theory in adults is that a natural vessel wall weakness is made worse by chronic sun exposure, hormonal changes, or injuries. The best ways to treat the problem at this time appear to be with lasers or laser-like pulsed-light therapy. No matter which modality is chosen though, care must be taken to ensure that the treatment and its results are better than the appearance of the original veins. In most people this is an isolated cosmetic problem and not part a greater medical condition. A scar on the face, even a small one, is much more noticeable than a small vein. Care in selecting an experienced physician and an appropriate treatment plan cannot be overemphasized.

WHAT PEOPLE LIKE YOU HAVE TO SAY

"After menopause, when the doctor put me on hormone replacement therapy, I started developing these tiny little veins on my face, especially around my nose and on my cheeks. I used to cover them with makeup, but I'm just getting tired of it. When I was younger, a doctor put a needle into a vein I had and gave it a little electric shock. It worked pretty well, but I just don't feel like having 20 or 30 electric shocks on my face. Can we use one of the lasers to treat this?"

Sarah V., age 54, a realtor and mother of one college-age daughter

Problem: Unsightly facial spider veins.

The Doctor's Recommendations: Laser-like pulsed-light therapy to treat all of the veins at one time.

Results: About three quarters of the veins were completely eradicated at one treatment session, in about a half an hour at the office. The other quarter required a second limited session, which lasted 15 minutes. The patient experienced redness over all the treated sites, some lasting until the next day. There was no bruising or scarring.

Total cost: $425 (a full session at $275 and limited session at $150). These costs are generally not covered by health insurance, but an occasional policy will reimburse for this treatment.

The Patient's Comments Post-Treatment: "I was a little disappointed that all the veins didn't go away the first time, but I was glad when they were completely gone the second. I had small red patches over all the veins that lasted until the next morning, and then they were gone. I thought this was much better than the needles stuck into my face with the electric shocks, which took much longer and left me with a little white crust over the vein that lasted about a week. The new way, I had no pain and no marks by the next day."

*

"Over the last few years, I have developed more and more veins on my cheeks and around my nose. It almost looks like I have been out drinking. It's starting to get embarrassing. What can we do to fix this problem?"

Bill K., age 61, a retired schoolteacher

Problem: Red spider veins on cheeks and nose, blue and purple veins on chin, red veins on chin.

The Doctor's Recommendations: Laser-like pulsed-light therapy to treat all the veins at once, but concern was raised over the difficulty of treating the blue-purple 1 mm facial and chin veins. These may require another treatment method in addition to pulsed-light therapy to completely clear.

Results: Complete clearance of all the red veins in 2 sessions. Unfortunately, minimal change occurred with the purple veins on the chin. Electrodesiccation was suggested, which the patient did not want it due to the possible complication of scarring. With reluctance, injection sclerotherapy was suggested for these isolated areas. Two limited sessions were needed to clear the purple veins.

Total cost: $700 (2 full pulsed-light sessions at $275 each, a limited sclerotherapy session at $150, and a last injection session to touch up remaining areas was done for free). These costs are generally not covered by health insurance, but an occasional policy will reimburse for these treatments. The patient developed some redness over the pulsed-light treated veins that resolved a few hours later. Mild bruising occurred at the injection sites that took about 1 week to resolve.

The Patient's Comments Post-Treatment: "We were unhappy that the purple veins didn't go away with the pulsed-light treatments the way the little red spider veins did. The doctor told us they may be harder to clear, but we just hoped it would work by itself. The needle sticks weren't bad, I just wish I didn't need to have them. It was nice that they didn't charge us for the last visit. But I am glad all the veins are now gone!"

CHAPTER 6

Leg Vein Blood Clots

WHAT ARE THESE?

A blood clot, or thrombus, can form in any of your leg veins. The depth of the clot (superficial or deep system), and the location of the clot (calf, thigh, or pelvis) can have a big effect on a person's short- and long-term recovery. The mere presence of a blood clot is a serious, sometimes life-threatening problem.

SUPERFICIAL BLOOD CLOTS

Blood clots in the superficial vein system are known as superficial thrombophlebitis. It is estimated that approximately 123,000 cases occur annually in the United States.[1] Unrecognized cases probably make the actual incidence even higher.[2] The exact cause of this problem is unknown. Several leading hypotheses include:

1. An irregularly shaped blood vessel allows blood to stagnate, leading to clot formation[3]
2. Direct injury to the vein wall[8]
3. Slow or blocked blood flow[8]

Most often there is no identifiable cause,[9] but it is a frequent complication of varicose veins.[4] The greater saphenous vein, the large vein that runs up the inside of the calf and thigh, is most frequently involved.

Symptoms can be similar to inflammation of the vein wall without a blood clot: There will be a dull ache in the affected region, sometimes

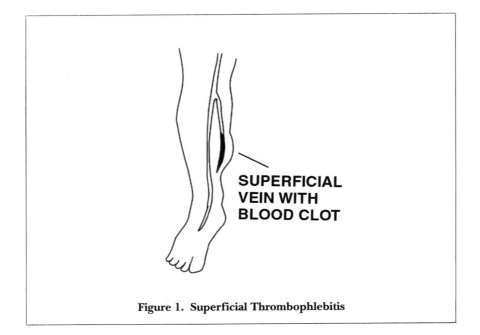

SUPERFICIAL VEIN WITH BLOOD CLOT

Figure 1. Superficial Thrombophlebitis

associated with some swelling of the calf or ankle, but swelling is more often an indication of a deep vein clot.[2] The skin overlying the vein can also be warm and tender if touched, and it certainly hurts when the affected area of the leg is squeezed.[3] Walking can cause pain and tenderness in the region of the involved vein. Often you can feel a hard cord along the length of the vein where the clot has formed. Some people also experience general fatigue, weakness, loss of appetite, and fever and chills. (Figure 1) If the clot extends to the junction with the deep system, a much more serious deep vein thrombosis may occur. Rarely a superficial blood clot can break off and go to the lung,[5,6] but this problem is far more common with deep vein blood clots.

Although most cases do not become severe enough to warrant treatment, it can at times produce significant problems. Symptoms generally last for a few days to a few weeks; occasionally they can persist for months.[7] Often thromboses will keep coming back. Sometimes this problem can affect the course of a nation. For example, Richard Nixon, during his presidency, was often troubled by this recurring disorder.

The diagnosis of superficial thrombophlebitis is usually straight-forward. People have pain along a cord-like vein, and there is usually redness and tenderness on exam. In the presence of varicose veins, the process is easy to identify. Without it, the diagnosis can be more challenging.[2] These cases often require the use of ultrasound testing to identify the presence and location of a clot.

TREATMENT OF SUPERFICIAL BLOOD CLOTS

As with all other diseases, prevention is the best therapy. Treatment for this problem depends on the location of the clot, how bad it is, and the underlying health of the patient. Many cases do not have obvious findings, and patients never obtain any form of therapy. Nonetheless, most of these patients fare quite nicely.

Patients who develop the previously described symptoms may require pain medicines. Aspirin is used to decrease the inflammatory response and mildly "thin the blood." An elastic compression stocking should be used to decrease the pain and control the swelling. Contrary to the age-old belief in the practice of bed rest and leg elevation, bed rest probably worsens the situation. It allows extension of the clot because the calf muscle pumps are not actively being used. Early use of the leg often hastens recovery. When pain and discomfort are incapacitating, moist heat packs and leg elevation, as well as the occasional use of stronger pain medication, are temporarily needed.

For many people symptoms last for 2 to 3 weeks. Swelling and redness, in addition to the discomfort, can also last this long. Careful follow-up with your physician may be required to insure resolution of the problem in a fast, uncomplicated fashion.

The role of surgery in superficial thrombophlebitis is unclear. Some advocate urgent removal of the localized clot if at all possible.[6] This may relieve the pressure on the blood vessel and more rapidly restore flow through it. Others feel that there is little indication for clot removal; the previously described treatment is all that is needed. However, if there is any evidence that the blood clot is moving up or out of the leg into the deep system or the pelvis, then surgical intervention to either remove the clot or tie off the greater saphenous vein in the groin to block its outflow would be indicated.[2,10]

When patients with varicose veins have persistent pain or frequently recurring clots, clear indications for surgical removal of the varicose veins exist.[2]

DEEP VEIN CLOTS

Blood clots in the deep veins of the leg, known as deep vein thromboses, can cause significant suffering and even death. It is a very serious problem affecting more than 2.5 million people each year in the United States alone.[11]

Leg pain is the most common complaint in deep vein thrombosis. Touching or squeezing the affected area makes it worse. There is also significant swelling of the limb in most patients. People are usually unable to walk on the leg due to the intense discomfort.

Deep vein blood clots occur most often below the knee. Fortunately, many of these can resolve completely without any long-term problems. When a clot moves up towards the trunk of the body however, or when it develops in the thigh or pelvic veins, much worse symptoms, complications, and long-term problems can occur.

Physical examination alone is usually not enough to diagnose a deep vein thrombosis; other tests are also needed. Until recently, the most useful test for diagnosing a blood clot was a venogram. For this test to be performed, the patient had to be transported to the radiology section of the hospital. A dye was then injected into a vein on the foot and allowed to travel back toward the heart. When a clot was present, the dye was unable to fill that vein. (Figure 2) Unfortunately, this test required moving some very sick patients to an area of the hospital where it was difficult to monitor them. Today, however, due to rapid advancements in the use of bedside duplex ultrasound, identification of blood clots in the deep venous system has become routine. This makes painful venograms unnecessary and allows treatment to begin sooner.

The most common cause for deep vein thrombosis is prolonged bed rest in patients with another illness.[3] It has been suggested that up to 70% of chronically ill patients may develop deep vein thromboses. In

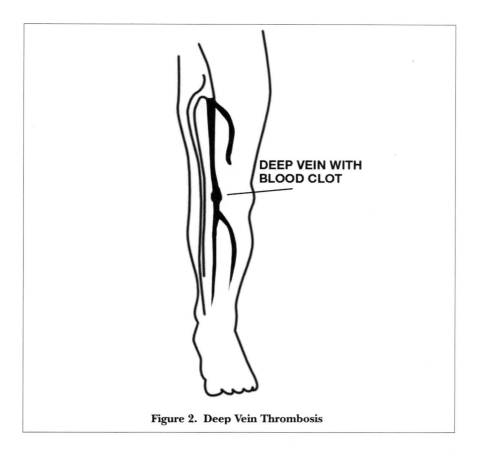

DEEP VEIN WITH BLOOD CLOT

Figure 2. Deep Vein Thrombosis

many people the initial finding may be a blood clot thrown to the lung.[3] Often patients with prolonged bed rest do not develop the significant leg swelling seen in active patients.

The other common causes for blood clots include:[3,11]

1. Advancing age
2. Slow blood flow, such as occurs during bed rest when the calf muscle pumps are not used to help return the venous blood to the heart
3. Infections
4. Age greater than 40
5. A recent heart attack
6. Congestive heart failure
7. A history of cancer

Other significant risk factors for the development of deep vein blood clots include:[3,11]

1. Obesity
2. Surgery, especially of the abdomen, hips, and pelvis
3. A previous history of deep vein thrombosis
4. Use of birth control pills

Even prolonged sitting such as taking a long car or plane ride can increase your risk. A recent French study documented that more than 4 hours of continuous travel during the 4 weeks before a deep vein thrombosis seems to be enough to increase the risk.[12] This study appears to conclusively confirm a suspicion that physicians have had for years that travel is associated with leg vein clot formation.

An unusual form of deep vein thrombosis can occur in women who have just given birth, called "milk leg." This term was originally coined from the mistaken idea that milk produced by nursing mothers eventually settled in their legs. But like other forms of deep vein thrombosis, it is a result of a blood clot. In this situation, the leg suddenly turns white, swells, and hurts. Otherwise it is similar to other deep vein blood clots.[3]

PREVENTING DEEP VEIN THROMBOSES

The best way to treat a deep vein thrombosis is to never let it happen. Once you've had it, the long-term effects are yours for life. There are two main approaches to preventing this problem.

The first method uses medication. Blood-thinning medicines are given as a preventive measure before the clot has a chance to form. This approach is frequently used in high-risk patients such as those who have had a previous deep vein thrombosis and those who have been placed in prolonged bed rest, following a major injury, illness, or surgery for instance. These medicines are also given before surgeries with a high incidence of postoperative deep vein clotting, such as hip replacements. Decreasing the risk of the blood clot far outweighs any danger from the slightly higher incidence of bleeding during surgery.

The other method does not use drugs. After surgery, childbirth, or injuries, elastic compression stockings, pumps that squeeze the blood out of your legs, leg elevation, and early walking are used. These techniques all use the calf muscle pump to propel the venous blood forward, preventing the slow flow and pooling of blood known to increase the chance of clot formation.

The approach used often depends on your doctor's preference, but certainly getting up and out of bed early, unless contraindicated for some important reason, is up to you, the patient. Getting up and moving around will, in general, make you feel better. By using your calf muscle pumps, you will decrease your risk for blood clot formation and a host of associated problems.

TREATMENT OF DEEP VEIN CLOTS

The treatment of deep vein clots has changed little over the past 30 years. The most common therapy used is blood-thinning medicine. Heparin, an intravenous blood thinner, is given in high doses to help your body dissolve the clot. It also prevents the clot from increasing in size. Patients with this problem, as opposed to those with superficial thrombophlebitis, are placed at bed rest. Bed rest gives deep vein clots a chance to attach themselves firmly to the vein wall, preventing pieces from breaking off and migrating to the lung when the patient walks on that leg.

Adequate blood thinning is critical for decreasing the chance of future deep vein clots. Too little thinning has been shown to produce a greater probability of repeat blood clots.[13] Some investigators have reported a fifteenfold increase in recurrent deep vein thromboses when the initial blood thinning was too low.[14]

A common cause for low initial treatment levels has been physician and patient concern with the bleeding risks associated with taking blood-thinning medicines. There is some validity to this concern, but only in special high-risk situations.[15] In most monitored patients, adequate and even high levels of blood thinning do not appear to be associated with an increased risk of important bleeding problems.[16]

Long-term patients are placed on warfarin pills, an oral anticoagulant, to prevent the formation of new clots and to help dissolve the old ones. This group of medicines interferes with the action of vitamin K, which is needed by your liver to make blood-clotting substances. They do not have an immediate effect; they generally require 3 to 5 days to work. Therefore patients need to be treated with intravenous heparin until warfarin takes effect.[16] Most people take these pills for 3 to 6 months after having a deep vein clot.

Monitoring of oral anticoagulation levels is critical. They can be too low or too high. If too low, long-term results will not be as good. If way too high, then major complications such as bleeding can occur. By adhering to the recommendations of your physician, most complications can be avoided.

Recently, the use of thrombolytic therapy, medications that very rapidly dissolve a clot, have come into vogue. Studies have shown that better long-term results can be obtained when these clot-dissolving medicines quickly reach the patient. A review of 13 studies found that about 45% of the patients treated in this fashion had significant or complete clearing on a post-therapy dye test. This compared to only 4% of those treated initially with intravenous heparin.[16] Thrombolytic agents also help to prevent leg swelling and help preserve vein valve function. The valves are critical to preserving normal blood return from a limb to the heart. Several studies have now shown that the majority of patients that were free from long-term leg problems had received thrombolytic therapy, whereas most of the patients with severe late leg conditions were treated with standard anticoagulants.[17,18]

These medicines, which are similar to the medicines given in an emergency by catheter to patients with heart attacks, have some problems. To directly administer the clot-dissolving medicine into the leg vein requires a significant technical ability not readily available in all hospitals. However, some studies have shown that by giving large amounts of large-clot-dissolving medicine anywhere in the bloodstream, a similar result may be obtained. Further studies are needed before this can be widely accepted in the medical community as a customary state-of-the-art therapy, but the early results appear to be excellent. It is a therapy we'll be hearing more about in the future.

Surgical intervention for deep vein thrombosis has very limited indications. The age of the blood clot certainly influences whether surgery can be effective. Doctors prefer to remove the clot if it is less than 2 to 3 days old, but diagnosis is often not made until later. Hence, there is little

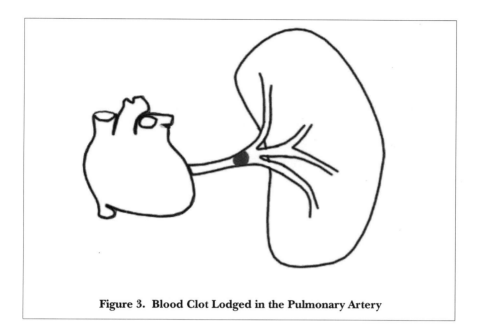

Figure 3. Blood Clot Lodged in the Pulmonary Artery

indication to see the surgeon. When used however, excellent short- and long-term results have been reported.[19,20] When compared to standard anticoagulation, the surgical patients often have a better outcome.

THE MOST DANGEROUS COMPLICATION

The worst complication associated with deep vein thrombosis is a blood clot thrown to the lung, known as a pulmonary embolism. This occurs when a clot or a portion of it breaks loose from the vein and travels through the bloodstream and through your heart, to lodge in the blood vessels to your lung. (Figure 3) When this happens, blood flow to that area is blocked, and you are suddenly unable to get oxygen into the blood being pumped to the rest of the body. When the clot is small in size, it may go unnoticed. However if it is large enough (and that size is different in each person), you can rapidly develop chest pain, shortness of breath, and cough. If the clot is massive, you are not able to pump an adequate amount of blood to stay alive, and rapid death can occur. The chest pain and shortness of breath lead to confusion with a heart attack, which can delay life-saving treatment by hours.

Blood clots to the lung are the third leading cause of death from cardiovascular disease, exceeded only by heart disease and stroke.[21] The exact number of deaths is unknown because most who die from this problem are never diagnosed.[24] The American Medical Association has estimated that 650,000 cases of pulmonary embolism occur in the United States each year.[3] Death occurs in approximately 30% of those patients. Physicians may miss 70% of the diagnoses in people who die of pulmonary embolism.[23] An additional 30% of those with non-fatal attacks will experience yet another pulmonary embolism.[3] It may be the most common preventable cause of death in hospitals.[22]

It is believed that approximately 90% of blood clots thrown to the lungs start in the legs.[3] At least 50% of the patients with symptomatic deep vein thromboses will have an asymptomatic pulmonary embolism.[24] Most blood clots develop in the calf veins and can spread upward into the deep veins of the thigh.[25] Because the clots in the thigh veins are larger, this location is more frequently associated with symptomatic pulmonary emboli.[26] But isolated calf blood clots are not harmless; many lead to blood clots that can break off and cause death.[27]

Diagnosis of this disorder can be difficult. A physical examination usually does not show any significant symptoms. An elevated heart rate may be the only sign. If a massive embolism occurs, there may be a large drop in blood pressure, but most of these patients do not survive long enough to have a diagnosis made. A measurement of the amount of oxygen in your bloodstream may also be performed, but again this is a nonspecific finding. Doppler ultrasound will frequently be ordered to see whether a clot is present in the leg. If so, the association will then be made that there was a pulmonary embolism because, as we previously stated, most pulmonary emboli originate from lower extremity blood clots.

The radiology tests used to diagnose this problem have changed over the last several years. In the past, a radioactive ventilation-perfusion scan was the primary test used. This study attempted to show where the blood was not actively circulating in the lungs, suggesting that a clot was present in that region. A dye study of the blood vessels to the lungs, called a pulmonary angiogram, was also performed. By injecting dye into the blood vessels of the lungs, a blood clot can be seen. These tests are now used less commonly due to advances in the ultrasound technique that allow bedside identification of a lower extremity clot. In the proper setting the association with a pulmonary embolism can then be made.[28]

TREATMENTS

Clot-dissolving medicines are the mainstay of therapy for pulmonary emboli. Intravenous heparin and long-term blood-thinning pills are used to treat patients. Most clots treated this way will dissolve over several days. Adequate anticoagulation has been shown to decrease the chance of repeat emboli to less than 5%.[22] Stronger clot-dissolving thrombolytic medicines are now commonly being used to treat this life-threatening problem. They appear to have promising early results, but only time will tell whether they will make a significant dent in the lives lost to this dreadful condition!

Surgery to remove clots from a lung is seldom performed. It is reserved for patients with massive embolization that have survived long enough for the diagnosis to be made. These are some of the sickest patients in the hospital, difficult to operate on because they are so unstable. But when the clot can be removed by surgery, a patient's medical picture can rapidly improve. As the stronger clot-dissolving therapy becomes more widespread, the indications for surgery will be even less frequent.

PREVENTION OF RECURRENT PULMONARY EMBOLI

Recently a filter or basket has been developed that can be placed in the inferior vena cava, the main blood vessel in the abdomen carrying the blood from the legs back to the heart.[29] Although these devices don't treat a clot already present in the lungs, they can catch pieces that may break off in the future. These filters are very effective for preventing large clots from reaching the lung and causing havoc. They have also been shown to decrease late death from additional pulmonary emboli.[29] Other indications for the filters include patients who cannot take blood-thinning medicines or have had a significant complication from them, failure of the anticoagulant (recurrent emboli), and people at high risk for developing a deep vein thrombosis. Examples of such patients include those with extensive injuries after an accident and those being prepared for a major orthopedic procedure.

The filters are made of materials that last virtually forever. They are placed either through the jugular vein in the neck or the femoral vein in the groin using local anesthesia. This has been a great advancement over previous filters that required major abdominal surgery, which sometimes led to a patient's death as rapidly as a pulmonary embolism.

LONG-TERM PROBLEMS AFTER DEEP VEIN BLOOD CLOTS

Chronic swelling is a common problem after a blood clot in the deep veins. Also, a constellation of findings called chronic venous insufficiency can develop. This is such a frequent problem that an entire chapter is devoted to it and the host of treatments available. Recurrent blood clots in the legs are also seen. Efforts to prevent these have already been discussed. The same holds true for recurrent blood clots to the lungs.

Simply using elastic compression stockings on a daily basis and attending to any changes in your legs may be the best thing anyone can do to protect themselves from future events.

SUMMARY

Blood clots in the legs are a common problem. They are a nuisance with mild discomfort at best, but more often they are a life-threatening problem. Different approaches are used to care for superficial and deep clots.

Superficial clots are easy to identify: There is pain and redness along a tender cord-like vein. The age-old approach, bed rest, probably worsens the situation because the calf muscle pumps are not utilized to push blood back to the heart. Walking, on the other hand, improves the situation and may hasten recovery.

Deep vein blood clots are a much more serious problem. The most common symptom is severe leg pain. People also develop significant swelling in the affected leg. Many clots occur below the knee. Some of these resolve without any problem, but most people are not that lucky, and long-term problems such as chronic venous insufficiency usually follow. When the clot extends upward toward the pelvis, or breaks off and goes to the lungs, this is an immediate life-threatening problem.

The diagnosis of a deep vein blood clot is based on a high degree of suspicion and the use of some tests. Bedside ultrasound of the leg veins has now become the most conclusive way to identify the problem and is now available in almost all hospitals.

Treatment of recent deep vein clots has always centered around blood-thinning medicines, which is first administered for several days through a peripheral skin vein. Patients are then given pills to take for about 3 to 6 months. Recently, rapid clot-busting medicines have been used to make clots dissolve more quickly. This may better preserve vein valve function, which when damaged is the probable cause for many of the long-term problems associated with a deep vein clot. With time, this will probably become the standard initial treatment for deep vein clots.

The worst complication of deep vein clots is a piece breaking off and going to the lungs. In many instances this life-threatening problem is the first sign that anything is wrong. The diagnosis can be difficult and time-consuming. Treatment usually centers around continuing the clot-dissolving medicines and trying to prevent further clots from reaching the lungs. Filters placed into the large vein in the abdomen have been developed to accomplish this goal. They catch the large pieces that do the most harm. Unfortunately, filters are usually placed after the first event; they do nothing for what has already happened.

Preventing clots from occurring is the best form of treatment. Two approaches are used in an attempt to prevent both first-time and repeat deep vein thromboses. The first method is based on medication. The second stresses early walking, and the use of elastic compression stockings following events such as childbirth, surgery, or an injury, using the calf muscle pump to empty the veins, thereby preventing blood from pooling in the legs and possibly causing clots. Clearly, avoiding the problem is the best option of all.

WHAT PEOPLE LIKE YOU HAVE TO SAY

"We had been traveling cross country for two weeks. On our way back I started developing severe leg pain. Then my leg started swelling. The last day in the car my calf hurt so much I didn't want to walk on it. After we got home and unloaded the luggage, I had my husband take me to the emergency room. They told me I had a blood clot."

Agatha P., age 62, a housewife, mother of five grown children and ten grandchildren

Problem: Deep vein thrombosis following prolonged sitting.

The Doctor's Recommendations: The patients venous ultrasound revealed she had a clot limited to her calf. It did not appear extensive enough to warrant catheter directed clot-dissolving agents such as urokinase, so she was admitted to the hospital, started on intravenous blood-thinning medicine, and then converted to pills. She had only mild swelling in her leg and was immediately placed in elastic compression stockings. She was able to resume walking on the third day after treatment. She remained on blood-thinning pills for 3 months and must wear her stockings lifelong. When traveling, she needs to get up every hour and walk around to help pump blood with her calf muscles.

Total cost: Less than $5,000. These charges should be covered by health insurance.

Results: Normal leg both in appearance and function.

The Patient's Comments Post-Treatment: "I thought at first the leg pain was just a muscle cramp. But when it didn't go away and my leg started swelling and I couldn't walk, I knew I was in trouble. Fortunately the doctors said it was only a small clot. They said my leg should be normal. I had always heard you needed to get up and walk around when on a long trip; I just didn't think it was that big a deal. I won't make that mistake again."

*

"They had problems taking my gallbladder out through the little scope, so they had to open me up. Instead of getting out of the hospital the next day, I spent 15 days there. The first time I got out of bed, 3 days after my surgery, I just collapsed. I had this sharp pain in my left chest every time I took a breath. I was really short of breath. They moved me to the intensive care unit. At first they thought I was having a heart attack, but then they said I was too young. Then they did a sound wave test on my legs. They found a blood clot and said that I had thrown a piece to my lungs."

Tammy K., age 29, a legal secretary, married, no children

Problem: Extensive deep vein thrombosis complicated by a pulmonary embolus.

The Doctor's Recommendations: Because of the location of the clot in her leg, the pulmonary embolism, and the recent surgery, she needed more than just blood-thinning medicine. She was taken back to the operating room, and under local anesthesia a filter was placed into the big abdominal vein that drained her legs and pelvis. Fortunately we were able to pass it up from the groin. Otherwise we would have had to stick it in through a vein in the neck. She was also started on blood thinner through her arm veins and was then converted to pills for the next 3 to 6 months. She was placed in elastic compression stockings with a recommendation that she wear them the rest of her life. This will decrease the risk of recurrent deep vein thrombosis and the development of the condition known as chronic venous insufficiency.

Total cost: Well in excess of $20,000 for the prolonged hospitalization, the intensive care unit stay, and the required surgeries. These charges should be covered by health insurance.

Results: She survived the life-threatening pulmonary embolus with no obvious long-term effects. Her leg looks pretty good after such an extensive blood clot. She will probably always have a little bit of swelling in that leg.

The Patient's Comments Post-Treatment: "I was really sick. The first week seemed like all kinds of things were happening.

The rest of the time they spent adjusting my blood-thinning medicine to get it to the right level. After about 3 days the pain in my side went away. Now that I'm home I don't want anything else to happen. I understand the need for the blood-thinning medicine and the blood tests. I just worry about the filter in my belly. They explained that it will last the rest of my life and that it has no real long-term complications, but it has only been around for 25 years no one knows what will happen after that! I know I need to wear my compression stockings. The doctors explained the possible problems if I don't. I hope I stick with them. Oh, well, I guess I'm just lucky to be alive."

CHAPTER 7

Chronic Venous Insufficiency: The Swollen Leg

Chronic venous insufficiency is a medical term used to describe a group of problems that can occur in diseased legs. These problems appear as a continuum of events that often takes up to 20 years to fully develop. The first stage is marked by swelling around the bone on the inside of your ankle, especially in the evening. Over time the skin begins to change color. The pigmentation often changes from a light color to dark brown as the red blood cells leak out of the blood vessel, and hemoglobin, the oxygen-carrying component of the red blood cells, stains the tissues. (Figure 1) Then a tired, heavy feeling develops in the legs,

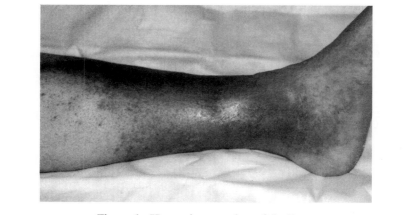

Figure 1. Hyperpigmentation of the Leg

the skin begins to get hard and thick, and areas of dermatitis (dry, flaky skin patches), redness, and inflammation occur. The leg can begin to itch and weep, and the swelling, which originally began around your ankle, can extend up the calf to the thigh. Finally, skin ulcers (open sores) can develop. (Figure 2) These may take months or even years to heal, only to reopen again at a later date. (Table I)

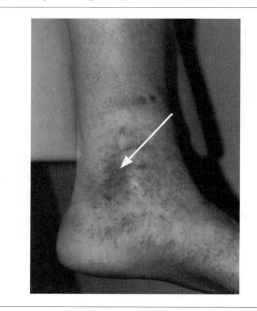

Figure 2. Open Venous Ulcer in a Patient Whose Only Risk Factor Was Untreated Varicose Veins.

Table I
Signs and Symptoms of Chronic Venous Insufficiency

Leg aches and pains

Night cramps

Ankle swelling

Dilated skin veins

Dense spider veins around the ankle

Pigmentation changes

Hardening and thickening of the skin

Skin inflammation

Weeping legs

Open sores

WHAT CAUSES IT?

Chronic venous insufficiency can result from a blood clot in the deep venous system. It has been estimated that up to 66% of those with deep vein thrombosis will develop this condition.[1] They will suffer with it their entire lifetime. But chronic blood clot blockages in the deep system do not seem to directly cause the problem. Apparently, secondary vein valve damage, leakage, and subsequent reflux are to blame.[1] Recent studies have found that 28 to 85% of patients with venous insufficiency may have leaky valves in the superficial veins or in combination with deep vein abnormalities.[2-4] To further complicate the picture, others have shown that longstanding varicose veins by themselves can cause these problems.[1,5] This complication takes many years to develop, and once it does, it requires lifelong care and treatment.

Your leg is in very poor condition if an open venous sore develops. Open sores require professional care and considerable lifestyle changes. Once healing is achieved, it is usually possible to maintain your leg in an acceptable condition by daily self-treatment, use of compression stockings, and frequent follow-up with your physician.

THE SCOPE OF THE PROBLEM

Severe chronic venous insufficiency is present in nearly 20% of working men and women.[6] It has been estimated that in the United States alone, more than 2 million workdays are lost each year due to complications from this condition.[7] Some of the lost work is the direct result of complications from untreated varicose veins. It has also been estimated that approximately 10% of those who suffer from chronic venous insufficiency wind up in the hospital at some time for treatment of a complication. Hence, this is not a matter to take lightly. If you have this problem, or think you have it, following some of the forthcoming suggestions may save you years of discomfort.

Studies have suggested that 1 to 2% of Western populations may have open venous ulcers at any one time.[8] This amounts to at least 500,000 people in the United States; most of them are women.[9] Some suggest that up to 1 million Americans are suffering from ulcers due to varicose veins.[10]

The cost for treating these ulcers in the United States is estimated to be $777 million to $1 billion per year.[11] In 1991, a Boston study calculated the cost of just outpatient visiting nurse care and supply charges, and found an overall cost of $1,900 per patient per month. This figure did not include any doctor visits, medications, antibiotics, nursing home charges, or needed hospitalizations, and did not consider whether the treatment was effective in healing the sore.[12] Since about 3% of the Medicare-age population has or has had an ulcer,[12] venous leg sores truly qualify as a costly public health problem.

Worldwide, the dollars spent on treating venous leg sores are even more staggering. In Germany for example, roughly 3.5 million people have chronic venous insufficiency, with some 1.2 million having developed venous leg ulcers. This translates to about $1.4 billion U.S. dollars per year in disability and direct treatment expenses for venous ulcers alone, in a country less than half the size of the U.S.[13] These findings seem to hold throughout the industrialized world.

TREATMENT

Elastic compression stockings are the mainstay of therapy for chronic venous insufficiency. Their exact mechanism of action is unknown. As previously described, stockings help prevent pooling of blood in the veins, which may improve the condition of the diseased vein valves and help the leg muscles pump venous blood. Another mechanism may be to directly decrease swelling. Together, these factors seem to improve the general well-being of the leg.

When venous ulcers develop, local wound care is also required. Bandages must be changed frequently, and a short course of oral antibiotics is common. Hospitalization is often needed if the sores are large and infected because intravenous antibiotics must be administered. Unfortunately, the success of local therapy is often inadequate. Complications from this problem are frequent.

In our experience, venous ulcers, if caught early, can be treated almost exclusively with local wound care and compression. We initially start with ace wraps and then convert to elastic compression stockings.

The treatment protocol used at our vein center includes:

1. Several days of bed rest with leg elevation either at home or in the hospital
2. Wound cleansing with soap and water followed by the application of bandages 3 times per day
3. Antibiotics for any signs of infection
4. Ace wrap compression, followed by elastic compression stockings when the frequency of dressing changes decreases
5. Moisturizing skin cream or occasionally steroid ointment on the surrounding areas of dry, scaly skin
6. Lifelong use of the compression stockings when the sores heal

The results of treating leg sores in this fashion have been quite good. Over 90% of the patients who faithfully wear the compression stockings can be healed.[14] Unfortunately healing time averaged longer than 5 months in most patients. Long-term results are also quite good. Sores came back in only 16% of the cases where patients wore the stockings daily, versus 100% of the cases where they would not.[14]

The major criticism of elastic compression therapy is that patients won't wear the stockings. But with today's advances in materials, texture, colors, and fit, this should no longer be a great concern.

A variety of kits with various medications, bandages, and special stockings have been developed to help treat longstanding, open sores. Many have decreased the time to heal the wound and aided the healing of some very difficult ulcers, but the mainstay of all the therapy is elastic compression stockings.

In and of itself, surgery, which usually involves wound cleaning and skin grafting, has not been very effective. But when varicose veins are identified alone, or in combination with, valvular leakage in the veins that connect the superficial and the deep systems, which is known as perforator incompetence, then surgery may be helpful. Aside from the varicose vein surgeries previously described, specific surgical procedures that divide the perforating veins and disconnect the low-pressure superficial venous system from the high pressures of the deep system are needed. This type of surgery, although effective in helping heal recurrent ulcers, has been marked by serious wound complications because incisions are often placed in swollen, heavily diseased tissue. Using new minimally invasive techniques though, complication rates have been significantly reduced. If these procedures are successful, the ulcers come back in less than 10% of the patients.[15]

TREATMENT SUMMARY

Compression stockings and local wound care can provide excellent results in managing chronic venous insufficiency and its worst complication, open sores. Unfortunately, it is a long and drawn-out affair, requiring months of effort to handle these terrible problems. Some patients may have open sores the rest of their lives. In these and a few other select patients, surgery to remove varicose veins and to divide incompetent perforator veins, if present, should be considered.

HELPFUL SUGGESTIONS

To help keep your legs in the best possible condition, before or after the diagnosis of chronic venous insufficiency is made, and before the onset of troublesome open leg sores, these guidelines may prove helpful:

1. Try to elevate your legs higher than the rest of your body a few times every day; keep your knees flexed since full knee extension may block full blood return to the heart. If possible, do activities such as reading lying down with your legs raised, rather than sitting at a desk.

2. Try to avoid prolonged standing or sitting without moving your legs. During long trips in a car, train, or airplane, move your feet often or get up for a walk. This helps the function of the muscular vein pump.

3. Take long walks whenever possible. While walking, wear your elastic compression stockings to improve the venous circulation. Although the elastic compression stockings alone do not pump the blood forward, they do decrease the amount of swelling that forms and do improve the blood flow during movement. To improve venous return to your heart, it has been shown that a long walk works better than just the activities of daily living.

4. Try to maintain your optimal body weight. Lose weight if necessary. Being overweight puts more strain on your legs and worsens the condition.

5. Stop smoking. Not only does smoking damage your heart and lungs, but it also affects your legs.

6. Pay attention to good foot and toenail care. Try to avoid any activities that may lead to injuries. Infections in a foot with chronic venous insufficiency are very difficult to treat. Wear comfortable shoes and avoid high heels. Dont walk barefoot.

7. If you suffer from dry skin, use a moisturizing cream. This helps prevent cracks from forming. Skin breaks can easily be infected by bacteria in a chronically diseased leg.

8. Put on your compression stockings early in the morning before you start your daily activities. This will prevent the swelling that develops as soon as you assume a standing position. Then, wear your stockings throughout the day. Whenever possible, bathe and shower in the evening, removing your stockings immediately beforehand. Then go to bed and elevate your legs.

9. Check your legs for swelling every evening. If you are in suitable compression stockings, your legs should not be swollen. If you find your legs swollen following the removal of the compression stockings, see your doctor and have the stockings replaced. In general, most elastic support hose will last 4 to 6 months. Replace the old support stockings when they wear out and lose compression. Remember to keep spare stockings on hand so you don't go for any length of time without needed support. Missing even a few days can significantly worsen your condition.

10. If any trauma or injury to your leg occurs, or if you begin to develop symptoms of swelling, itching, redness, pain, or fever, contact your physician immediately. If not rapidly treated, small and apparently trivial injuries can become serious problems, often leading to a large open sore. When caught early, these can often be aggressively managed, limiting their size and the time needed for their care.

11. Treat vein problems such as varicose veins early in their course before complications occur. With so much new data demonstrating that untreated varicose veins by themselves may lead to the horrors of chronic venous insufficiency and longstanding open sores, a few hours of treatment can save years of misery.

WHAT PEOPLE LIKE YOU HAVE TO SAY

"After the birth of my last child I developed milk leg. My leg started hurting. Then it started swelling. It hurt so much I couldn't stand on it. At first I thought I had milk lodged in my leg. Only later did I understand that this was from a blood clot. They started me on blood-thinning medicine through my arm veins and then switched me to pills. I wasn't able to breast-feed my son because the medicine could have passed through my milk and harmed him. Anyway, for 3 months I had to take those pills. Once each week I had to get a blood test done to make sure my blood wasn't getting too thick or too thin. Finally I was able to stop them. For years this leg has been a little more swollen than the other. Over the last 5 years it also started getting a brown discoloration over the shin. Now it has dry flaky skin. Is there anything special I need to do to stop this from getting worse? Am I going to have any other problems?"

Sally McK., age 67, a housewife, mother of three grown children, with two grandchildren

Problem: Previous lower extremity deep vein thrombosis, now with chronically swollen leg and findings of chronic venous insufficiency.

The Doctor's Recommendations: Since the immediate effects of the blood clot have long been treated, the main emphasis now should be to prevent any recurrent clots or long-term complications. The patient should be fitted with elastic compression stockings and should wear them lifelong. They will help decrease the chronic swelling and help avert some of the problems associated with chronic venous insufficiency. She needs to put them on first thing in the morning, wear them all day, and take them off at night before going to sleep. She should routinely check the skin of her affected leg to look for any changes or signs of an early infection. Walking is also an effective preventive measure. She needs to develop a program and faithfully follow it. This will help the calf muscle pumps increase venous return to the heart. If she is in an accident, placed at prolonged bed rest for any reason, or has major surgery in the future, she must tell her doctors about her previous blood clot. They can use blood-thinning medicine, pneumatic compression stockings, or both to help prevent another clot from forming. When she goes on a long trip, she should get up periodically and walk around. If she starts developing any significant leg pain or an increase in the amount of swelling, she needs to quickly see her doctor. She may be developing another clot. The dark brown pigmentation change is permanent, but early attention to the other skin changes of dermatitis may decrease the likelihood she will develop inflammation, fluid weeping from the skin, recurrent infections, and possibly open sores. Elevating her legs several times a day may also help drain some of the edema fluid, but the mainstay of treatment at this time is the use of elastic compression stockings.

Results: Stabilization of her condition and avoidance of open venous leg ulcers.

Total cost: It is hard to estimate since this is a lifelong battle. If the skin can be kept from breaking down and getting infected, then only periodic office visits will be needed. Generally they would need to occur every 3 months at about $50 per visit, which comes to about $200 per year. In most cases these are covered by health insurance or, as in this case, Medicare. Two pairs of panty hose elastic compression stockings will be needed at about $120 per pair (1 to wear and 1 to wash), which must be replaced about every 6 months (4 pairs per year). Usually, these are covered only partially or not at all by insurance plans.

In a best-case scenario, the cost per year is about $600. The sky is the limit if complications such as infections and ulcers develop. These problems may generate costs in areas such as antibiotics, frequent office visits, home nursing for wound care, and hospitalizations.

The Patient's Comments Post-Treatment: "I wish they would have told me to wear the compression stockings years ago. I was so scared I would have done anything. Now I have this swollen leg with a large brown patch on it. The skin feels woody and it's always scaling, even when I use moisturizing lotion. All I do is worry that I'll develop an open sore. I would gladly have worn the stockings. At first they're hard to get on, but after a while your legs feel funny without them. Maybe I could have avoided the swelling, the pigmentation changes, and the hard thick skin up and down my shin."

*

"When I was 19, I was in a bad car accident. I fractured my pelvis and developed a bad blood clot in the vein in my belly that drained my left leg. They treated me with blood-thinning medicines for months. Finally I was able to get off of them. I've had two children. Fortunately I didn't get another clot with the pregnancies. But each time my leg has gotten a little more swollen. Over the last 10 years the skin around the inside of my ankle has gotten dark brown. For the last 5 years I keep developing these painful sores that break open. Usually they heal, but this one has been open for 6 months. Once somebody tried a skin graft to the area. It only worked for a short time and then the ulcer opened up again right in the middle of it. Every time the sore opens up, it's real painful. They put me at bed rest with my leg elevated. That's not so bad now, but it was terrible when my kids were little. Sometimes they say its infected and start me on some expensive antibiotics. Fortunately my husband is willing to help me with the bandage changes. We used to have the nurses come to the house, but that's really expensive and my insurance only covered a small amount. The biggest problem though is I end up missing a lot of work and pay. I work at the cosmetics counter and so I stand all the time. When my sores break open, I can't work. For years I refused to wear the elastic support stockings because I thought they were ugly. Now they say I'm paying for it. I wear them every day now, even when I have a sore. What can I do now to try and prevent even more problems?"

Kim R., age 37 a retail sales clerk, housewife, and the mother of two school-age children

Problem: Previous very extensive iliac vein deep vein thrombosis. She now has a chronically swollen leg and the skin findings of chronic venous insufficiency. This has progressed to the point of recurrent ulcer formation.

The Doctor's Recommendations: The main emphasis now is to heal her open leg sores and try to prevent their recurrence. We have started her on 3-times-a-day dressing changes in an effort to keep the wound clean and allow the skin to heal in from the edges. Many methods of treating these wounds have been developed. In our experience cleansing with good-old soap and water works best. A venous ultrasound should also be performed to look for perforator vein incompetence in the area of the sore. If it is present, then a surgical procedure to tie off the leaking veins needs to be considered. Otherwise the wound will tend to keep breaking open above the incompetant valve. In this case the veins did not show significant valvular leakage in this area, so surgery was not indicated. She also did not have varicose veins which we could remove to help heal the wound.

This patient was treated only with oral antibiotics and dressing changes. Ace wraps were initially used for compression on her legs so the dressing changes would be easier. Once the wound started to heal, she was placed in standard elastic compression stockings, and she has agreed to wear them daily instead of occasionally, as she did previously. She needs to put them on first thing in the morning and wear them all day; then take them off at night to bathe and sleep. The brown pigmentation changes on her shin and ankle are permanent, but many of the other skin changes can be controlled with good care. A daily walking program was outlined to increase venous return via the calf muscle pumps. If she starts developing any increase in swelling, redness, or skin changes, she needs to immediately see a doctor because she may be on the verge of developing another ulcer, and aggressive early treatment may limit its size and severity. She should elevate her legs several times every day in an effort to decrease some of the edema fluid. She should also consider changing her job to one that does not require her to stand all day, thereby decreasing the pressure from gravity and her body weight on the healing wound. Unfortunately, this will be a lifelong problem.

Results: The open venous ulcer healed after several months, and there is good control of the progression of the chronic venous insufficiency. If she continues to wear her compression stockings the ulcer recurrence rate will be decreased. Unfortunately, she will never have a completely normal leg.

Total cost: It is hard to estimate since this is a lifelong problem, and it is impossible to predict how many leg ulcers she will develop. As with the previous case, if recurrent skin ulcers can be prevented, then only periodic office visits will be needed, generally every 3 months at about $50 per visit, or about $200 per year. These are generally covered by health insurance or Medicare. Two pairs of panty hose elastic compression stockings will be needed at about $120 per pair (1 to wear and 1 to wash), which must be replaced about every 6 months (4 pairs per year). These are usually covered only partially or not at all by insurance plans. In a best-case scenario the cost per year is about $600. If she continues to develop recurrent venous ulcers, there is no way to predict how high the costs may go. Expenses to consider are antibiotics, frequent office visits, home nursing for wound care, and possibly hospitalizations. Also, you need to factor in lost wages from missed work and possible childcare. All told, it's much better to prevent the problem than to try and treat it.

The Patient's Comments Post-Treatment: Every time my leg heals, I think this is the last time it will happen. Then 4, 5, 6 months later, it will break open again. Then we start the process all over again. I wish I would have worn the support stockings the first day after my car accident. Maybe I would have never gotten into this mess."

CHAPTER 8

Arm Vein Blood Clots

Blood clots in the deep arm veins are not common. They account for less than 2% of all significant vein thromboses.[1] Until recently it was believed that this problem had few long-term effects; however this conclusion was generated from a limited amount of information. Furthermore, many of the initial studies were based on young, otherwise healthy people. We now know that when arm vein clots are left untreated, up to 75% of the patients will have some long-term limitations,[2,3] up to 12% will throw a blood clot to their lung, and up to 1% of patients will die.[4,5] Hence, this is now considered a serious problem.

THE CAUSES

Most frequently, arm clots are caused by an abnormal first rib pushing on the deep veins that drain the arm (Paget-Schrotter Syndrome), by frequent repetitive arm activities such as weight lifting or push-ups (effort thrombosis), and by catheters placed into arm veins for the long-term administration of chemotherapy, nutrition, and monitoring. With approximately 500,000 catheters inserted each year in the United States alone, this is now becoming the most frequent cause of arm blood clots.[6] Three percent of the patients with these catheters, or about 15,000 patients each year, will develop significant arm vein clots.[7] Thousands more will have clots not severe enough to warrant aggressive treatment. (Figure 1)

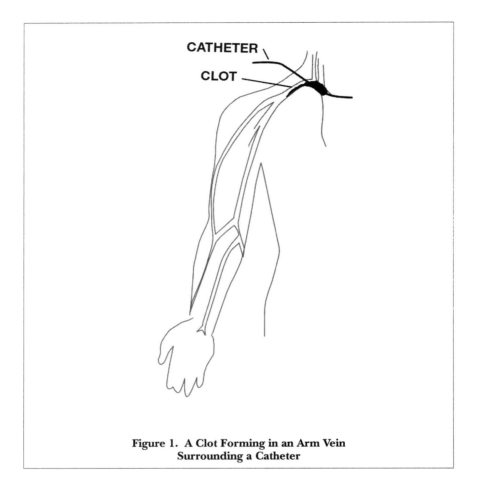

CATHETER

CLOT

Figure 1. A Clot Forming in an Arm Vein Surrounding a Catheter

THE FINDINGS

Most patients have a sudden onset of massive swelling. Varying degrees of pain, discomfort, and loss of arm motion can be present as well. On examination, there is usually tenderness overlying the involved vein and a blue discoloration of the arm. Occasionally you can feel a cord-like structure, which is the clot. The arterial pulse in the wrist is often decreased due to the extensive swelling. These symptoms may last for days or weeks as the body looks for new ways to drain the blood out of your arm. Blood clots can occur again and again with inadequate treatment. Fortunately, limb loss is rare.

DIAGNOSIS

The diagnosis of deep vein thrombosis of the arm can usually be made from a patient's history and a physical examination. Doppler ultrasound identifies the exact site of the clot, and venography, injecting dye into the vein, can confirm the location and will outline the clot.

TREATMENT

Primary therapy for this problem is heparin, a blood-thinning medicine. It is followed long term by blood-thinning pills. If pulmonary emboli occur or when blood-thinning medicine is not appropriate, placing a filter into the superior vena cava is indicated, just as filters are placed in the inferior vena cava for catching lower extremity blood clots. It appears that a high incidence of blood clots to the lungs can be documented in patients with arm clots.[8]

With moderate success, many hospitals have also started to use the strong clot-dissolving medicines for arm clots. This resolves the clot more rapidly and leaves the patient with less disability.

If the cause for the obstruction is identified, it should be treated. For instance, if catheters are present, they should be removed from the vein. When an abnormal first rib causes a vein blockage, surgical removal of the rib is indicated to prevent recurrence. (Figure 2) This surgery is extremely well tolerated and allows definitive removal of the cause for obstruction.

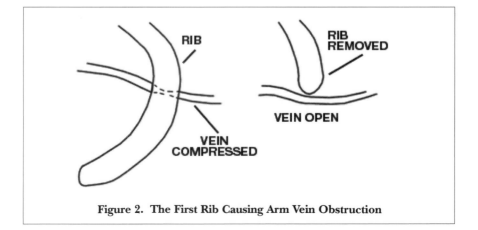

Figure 2. The First Rib Causing Arm Vein Obstruction

LONG-TERM PROBLEMS

The most serious long-term problem with this condition is a chronically swollen arm. In some cases the arm becomes so massive that it cannot be used. The appropriate treatment for this particular problem is similar to the treatment for blood clots in the leg. Special elastic compression sleeves and in some cases full upper-body compression jackets have been designed for patients with this condition. Most patients can also benefit from upper extremity pneumatic compression devices that act just like the similar devices for the leg—in this case, they squeeze fluid out of the arm to make it useful again.

SUMMARY

A recent review of the literature has shown a shift from reports of young patients with effort vein thrombosis to increasing numbers of elderly patients with central venous catheters or cancer presenting with upper extremity deep vein blood clots. Arm clots are diagnosed from the patients history and a clinical examination. Confirmation is by an ultrasound test. Dye tests can also be used.

Treatment is with blood-thinning medicines. Surgery is occasionally performed as well. If left untreated, 75% of those with arm clots end up with a chronically swollen arm with limited function.

WHAT PEOPLE LIKE YOU HAVE TO SAY

"I don't know which is worse—my mastectomy, my hair falling out from the chemotherapy, or now my arm always being swollen from the blood clot around the catheter? I think the swelling is worse. It got a little better after they took the catheter out, but not by much. It hardly ever goes down and I can barely use my arm. At least I could wear a wig."

Pat D., age 67; retired after her surgery, she is the primary caregiver for her ill husband. There are no other family members to help.

Problem: A massively swollen arm from a clot in the main vein that drains blood from the arm. The clot formed around the catheter placed in it for administering chemotherapy.

The Doctor's Recommendations: This is a very difficult, life-long problem. An attempt was made to use thrombolytic therapy, but it did not work. The patient was therefore placed on intravenous heparin and then oral warfarin to help dissolve the clot. Since her arm was very swollen, it was ace wrapped and kept elevated all the time hanging from a pole. This helped to decrease the swelling. A pneumatic compression sleeve was then used to help squeeze as much fluid as possible from the arm. When the size of her arm stabilized, she was measured and fitted for a custom elastic compression sleeve that started at her wrist and went up and over her shoulder. When her swelling worsens, she will have to use the pneumatic compression device at home. She will have to wear the elastic compression sleeve the rest of her life to have any hope of keeping the fluid down so that she can use her arm. She must wear it all day long, taking it off only to bathe and sleep. At night she must prop her arm up on two pillows to keep the swelling down. After 3 and then 6 months, attempts were made to discontinue the blood-thinning pills, but both times her swelling worsened, so the pills were resumed. She should take them for the rest of her life.

Total cost: The initial hospitalization was well in excess of $15,000. These charges should be covered by health insurance or, as in this case, Medicare. The remaining cost is hard to estimate since this is a lifelong problem. Two pairs of custom elastic compression sleeves are generally about $250 (1 to wear and 1 to wash). They are replaced about every 6 months (4 pairs per year). This patient must also rent or purchase a pneumatic compression device and periodically replace the plastic sleeves that attach to the machine. She will also be on blood-thinning pills the rest of her life, will require periodic blood tests, and will occasionally need doctors office visits. These costs are usually covered partially or not at all by most insurance plans. If any further hospitalizations are required, costs will increase dramatically.

Results: Her arm is always moderately swollen, but she can still use it.

The Patient's Comments Post-Treatment: "This is your worst nightmare! My arm is always swollen and it blows up like a balloon if I don't wear the sleeve. If I don't elevate my arm a couple of times during the day, by evening the sleeve gets real tight and my hand gets puffy. I tried to stop wearing the elastic glove for my hand swelling but if I don't, I can't do anything. At least they've got it to the point where I can use my arm most of the time. Unfortunately, they had to move the catheter to the other side to give me my chemotherapy. I hope that side doesn't clot as well. Then I don't know what I would do."

*

"I was lifting some weights at my health club. Usually I just do aerobics, but this time I thought I would do some strength training as well. Suddenly I got this severe pain in my shoulder. My arm started swelling and turned blue. I went straight to the emergency room. They gave me a shot since I was in so much pain. Then they did a sound wave test and told me I had a blood clot in my arm. I thought, How is this possible, I'm only 24 years old?

"They started me on blood-thinning medicine through my vein and had this chest surgeon see me. I was really scared. He had the radiologist do a dye test. They stuck this catheter in from a vein in my groin and ran it up to my arm. It showed a blood clot in my arm. I was scared to death!"

Mitzie S., age 24 a single legal secretary

Problem: A massively swollen arm from a clot in the main vein that drains the arm, which developed after repetitive weight lifting.

The Doctor's Recommendations: Mitzie presented early with this problem. By history and examination we were fairly sure of the diagnosis. We started her on blood-thinning medicine and got an ultrasound to make sure there were no surprises. It documented the clot. We then had the radiologist do a dye test, which confirmed the thrombus blocking the main vein that drains her arm. Thrombolytic agents were used and the clot dissolved. We then did another dye test and it showed that the tip of the first rib was compressing the vein. We recommended surgery and took out the rib without difficulty. The dye test was repeated and it showed a small area of residual narrowing in the vein, the result of some scar tissue from the rib irritation. The radiologist was able to stretch this area open using a balloon catheter. We kept her on blood-thinning pills for 3 months, and then discontinued the pills. She did not need an elastic compression sleeve or long-term ace wraps.

Total cost: In excess of $20,000.00 for the hospitalization, radiology procedures, and surgery. She required blood-thinning pills and periodic blood tests, which were discontinued after 3 months. These charges should be covered by health insurance.

Results: She has a normal arm, no swelling, and no limitations.

The Patient's Comments Post-Treatment: "At first I didn't know what to expect. Things were happening so fast. When they got the clot dissolved, the swelling really started going down. I didn't want surgery, but I really didn't want this to happen again! I'm a little sore from the operation, but I'm thankful I have a normal arm. I didn't know what would happen when it started swelling, hurting, and turning blue."

CHAPTER 9

Don't Worry!

"I get so tired of people telling me, 'It's no big deal, it's only varicose veins.' Sometimes my legs hurt so much I can hardly stand. Then they tell me it's cosmetic. My insurance company won't pay for anything to be done because I haven't had a complication yet! They want me to wait until I get an open sore or the veins start bleeding. Some policy I have. Next they'll tell me I can't have a mammogram until I have breast cancer or an EKG until I have a heart attack. I don't have the money to pay for any of this out of pocket. It gets me so down. I just don't know what I am going to do!"

WHAT IS DEPRESSION?

Depression, as defined in *Stedman's Medical Dictionary,* is a "descriptive syndrome for a cluster of symptoms and features commonly occurring in middle life and in the absence of precipitants." It is associated with severe mood changes and often decreased ability or interest in performing the functions of daily life such as bathing, cleaning, and eating. It varies in severity during the day, often being worse in the morning. Sufferers can awaken from sleep too early and have insomnia in the middle of the night. Weight loss, guilt, and lack of interaction with the environment are common, and it can also be associated with a reaction to an intensely sad situation such as the loss of a loved one or very good friend. During depression, one can have sinking spirits, dejection, apathy with feelings of melancholia, and indifference to the surroundings. It can also lead to sluggish and painful thought processes. This is a real medical problem and can be a medical emergency if suicidal thoughts develop from the helplessness and hopelessness. But fortunately, most people don't have clinical depression! Like migraines and asthma, it's a commonly-used term that more people claim to have than really do.

IF I DON'T HAVE DEPRESSION, WHAT DO I HAVE?

Most of us experience periods of being down in the dumps, most often as a reaction to unpleasant events at home or at work. We usually label these feelings the "blahs" or the "blues." Feeling unhappy when bad things occur, such as the loss of a job or an argument with a loved one, is a normal reaction. We feel bad for several days or possibly weeks, and then we return to our normal emotional state of good health. The problem arises when these feelings linger indefinitely or are blown out of proportion relative to the importance of the troubling event. In those cases more help than just a comforting word or a shoulder to lean on may be required.

HOW CAN I DISTINGUISH BETWEEN THE BLAHS AND THE REAL THING?

Periodically, everyone has symptoms of depression, but they go away in an appropriate period of time. We all face stressful situations over love, work, or money that push us to the limit, but somehow we keep going. However, when you no longer see the light at the end of the tunnel, when the symptoms totally consume you, when you are no longer able to perform the daily functions of life and the feelings drag on for weeks or longer or you are thinking about ending it all, then you should definitely see your doctor. Of course you can see your doctor at any point along the way. It's just that when life becomes too troubling to bear, rapid medical intervention through counselling, medications, or other treatments are needed. Some of the more serious symptoms that require attention are:[2]

- Thoughts of dying or suicide
- Feelings of worthlessness and hopelessness

- Inability to sleep or sleeping too much
- Nightmares
- Always feeling fatigued
- New aches and pains not related to any true medical condition
- New headaches not related to any true medical condition
- Difficulty concentrating or remembering things
- Uncontrolled anxiety
- Low self-esteem
- Loss of interest in sex
- Loss of interest in things you normally enjoy
- Increased irritability
- Weight swings

These are just some of the more common findings; there are many more symptoms of depression, so don't use this list to ignore, diagnose, or treat yourself! True depression is not a matter to take lightly. Only qualified medical professionals can tell you what's going on. Seek their advice without delay! If you can't afford treatment, call your county health department. Almost all of them offer free or reduced-rate mental health clinics that are within the reach of everyone's pocketbook.

HOW DO VEIN PROBLEMS FIT IN?

Many people with varicose veins and other chronic vein disorders feel down in the dumps about their problems. People with open leg sores can develop genuine depression due to the long-term nature of the problems. But good news—treating your vein problems can often help those other problems as well.

WHO IS AT RISK FOR DEPRESSION?

Certain groups of people are more prone to depression than the general population:[2]

- Those with a chronic medical condition such as lower extremity blood clots, swelling, or open leg sores
- Women
- Those previously treated for real depression
- Those whose first depressive event occurred before 40 years old

- Those who have attempted suicide
- Those who abuse alcohol or drugs
- Those who have a family history of depression
- Those who have recently had a major life change
- Those who have little or no support system
- Those who have recently had a baby

Just because you have one or more of these risk factors doesn't mean you will have a problem with depression. This list simply indicates those who have a higher risk than others. In addition, this list is not complete. It's provided as a springboard to encourage those who may need treatment to seek help.

TREATMENT FOR DEPRESSION

Today, most doctors attack depression from several angles—medication, therapy, and stress reduction. These complex treatments are beyond the scope of this book, but some generalities can be touched on.

Antidepressant drugs have markedly decreased the need for hospitalization and other forms of therapy such as the electroshock treatments that were still frequently in use when we were medical students. Although it may take several weeks to work, long-term drug maintenance is safely possible for those who need it. This often prevents recurrent episodes.

Therapy, often through counseling and support groups, has had great success in treating both mild and chronic depression. Unfortunately, we are unaware of specific support groups for some of the more problematic vein problems, such as arms or legs that are chronically swollen from blood clots or the recurring nightmare of an open venous leg ulcer. But in general, help is available at both the individual and group levels within driving distance for virtually everyone in America today.

Stress reduction has become a topic of great interest since everyone faces some stress every day. But the way it affects each individual varies, as do the effective coping mechanisms. Bookstores and libraries have shelves lined with suggestions on how to do it. Even television infomercials give testimony to various methods that may work. We suggest that whatever works for you is the best method. Just because a technique doesn't have a well-known sponsor doesn't mean it's wrong.

Some universal stress reduction techniques include:[2]

- Get a good night's sleep
- Eat a well-balanced diet
- Get plenty of exercise
- Use alcohol in moderation if you drink, and try to avoid it just before bedtime
- Pace yourself to get the required tasks completed
- Follow a regular daily activity schedule
- Don't take on more than you can get done at home, work, or play
- Set aside time to unwind and relax each day
- When your medical conditions are a problem, cut back activities to allow for more rest
- Get professional help when you or others feel you need it

You can beat the blahs, the blues, and depression! Don't give in to the problems and complications of vein disease, or to a host of other medical problems from arthritis to heart disease for that matter. First, have a positive attitude. This may sound corny, but those who do seem to fair much better than those that don't. To steal a phrase from the 1960s civil rights movement: we shall overcome. Or better yet: you shall overcome. All it takes is the right mindset, treating problems rapidly when they arise, picking qualified, interested people to help you with your condition, seeking professional and spiritual help whenever needed, and most of all, remembering that you are not alone.

CHAPTER 10

What You Can Do to Help Yourself

Although you cannot completely prevent vein problems, there are many common sense things you can do to influence the severity of their symptoms. You may even prevent some conditions from occurring. If you already have vein problems, following some simple suggestions may lessen their impact or help prevent some of the more serious and possibly life-threatening complications. You can never know for sure, and no one can ever guarantee, that when these simple things are done, problems won't develop, but at least you'll have the peace of mind of knowing you tried to prevent them. Somehow, that alone seems to take some of the sting out the situation. Before making any significant lifestyle changes though, always consult your doctor, since he or she may be able to help select a plan or approach that's right for you.

Now let's take a look at some of the more common things you can do with little to no significant change in your daily activities.

DIET

As with all other health-related conditions, you must remember that you are what you eat. The role of diet is not as clear-cut in vein disorders as it is for problems such as heart disease, breast cancer, and diabetes, but there appears to be certain common patterns.

Your colon, also known as your large intestine, is the final repository of fecal matter prior to defecation. Low-fiber diets play a role in the development of hard stools and chronic constipation. This forces the individual to strain on bowel movements leading to an increase in pressure in the belly. In Great Britain, doctors have suggested that this pressure is transmitted to your leg veins, thereby causing them to dilate. After a while the valves malfunction and subsequently varicose veins develop. This process doesn't take place overnight, but is the culmination of years of poor eating habits. Additionally, it is thought that the colon itself may press on the pelvic veins, mildly obstructing the drainage of these veins, which also could lead to a backup of pressure in the system.[2]

Fiber seems to decrease the transit time of stool through the colon, keeping it light and bulky rather than hard and small. Fiber, also known as roughage, is commonly found in grains, beans, peas, and many nuts. Low-fiber foods include meat, fish, eggs, dairy products such as milk and cheese, processed sugar, and alcoholic beverages.

A low-fiber diet has been associated with the development of varicose veins.[1] Although this is not a cause-and-effect relationship, a simple change to more fiber may alleviate the severity of a problem or delay its onset. It may also decrease your risk for diseases like diverticulitis, diverticulosis, and colon cancer.

Limiting your intake of fat may also help with varicose vein problems. Since fats are high in calories, they can significantly add to your waistline, leading to more weight on the veins of your legs. Also, some fatty acids, the breakdown products of fats in your bloodstream, have been shown to directly cause inflammation, which may make phlebitis worse in select individuals. Other fatty acids have been shown to directly stimulate the development of blood clots.[10-12]

Eat a well-balanced diet high in nutrients and vitamins. Although we don't know for sure how most vitamins are involved in vein problems, we do know that a lack of them is a problem. In an effort to combat the problem of vitamin deficiencies, the United States government has advocated the addition of many of these to our diet, vitamin D in milk, and thiamine and niacin (B complex vitamins) in flour and breads for example.

The role of vitamin C and zinc in wound healing is now fairly well accepted. They appear to be directly involved in growth and repair. Some physicians give additional amounts of these supplements when facing big, open, leg sores. On the other hand, others feel that if you eat right, you get more than enough of these necessary nutrients.

Most of all, use common sense when taking vitamin and mineral supplements. A well-balanced diet usually provides all the vitamins, minerals, and nutrients your body needs to perform the normal activities of daily living. A little can go a long way. Only one ounce of vitamin B12, a common supplement, can supply the estimated daily requirement of this vitamin for about 4 million people.[3] So use moderation and don't overdose on supplements. Too much of a good thing can be harmful to you and even your family. An estimated 2,000 children in the United States each year are poisoned by accidentally taking their mother's iron supplements.

WATCH YOUR WEIGHT

Being overweight directly increases the pressure on your legs. This can lead to increased vein pressure, which can contribute to the development or worsening of varicose veins. Also, increased pressure can significantly worsen venous stasis changes that may be present.[13]

If you are overweight, try to lose pounds in a sensible fashion. Avoid fad diets. Most people on these diets take off pounds and inches quickly, but when the novelty wears off, they frequently put more weight back on than they originally lost, leading to an overall net gain in weight. The reason seems to be that the lifestyle modifications and proper dietary habits that keep the pounds off have not been learned. Overweight people succumb to the get-rich-quick scheme, or in this case the get-pounds-off-quick plan. Unfortunately fad diets seldom lead to long-lasting results. If you need help accomplishing your goals, seek the advice of your physician, a registered dietician, or a professional weight loss center to structure a safe diet plan that is right for you.

STOP SMOKING

Smoking has been linked to or blamed for all sorts of diseases and cancers. So a recommendation to stop smoking for vein problems should come as no surprise. But specifically for women who smoke *and* take birth control pills, the findings are even stronger.

For a time, it was thought that the problem of superficial blood clots was related only to the high hormone concentrations found in the early birth control pills, because as the dosages decreased, so did the number of strokes and heart attacks associated with them. But the amount and kinds of estrogen present are not sufficient to explain all vein problems. Although higher estrogen means more clots, and lower estrogen means less clots, it has not been definitively shown that the pill alone is to blame. Smoking appears to play a big role.

Studies have shown that women who smoke and take even low-dose estrogen pills have a greater risk of vein thrombosis than nonsmokers.[4] This alone should be enough motivation to stop anyone from smoking.

Smoking also impedes wound healing. This can be important for people trying to heal leg sores, and is especially significant for women who also have hardening of the arteries. Nicotine seems to cause constriction of the blood vessels, further impeding blood flow in an area that already has compromised circulation. Smoking also directly decreases the concentration of oxygen in the bloodstream, compounding an already bad problem.

CONSIDER AN ASPIRIN A DAY

Most of the information on the effects of aspirin have come from studies on men, but many studies are now showing similar results in women. Most of the work has been done on heart disease, where aspirin has been shown to decrease the incidence of recurrent heart attacks and death. The mechanism is thought to be based on aspirin's ability to prevent blood clots in the small coronary arteries that supply the heart muscle proper. Similar anti-clotting effects may in time be proven in veins as well. At least one major study supports this conclusion.[5] Remember, check with your doctor first, but a single aspirin a day may turn out to play a significant role in preventing blood clot formation throughout your body.

EXERCISE AND WALKING

As we get older, we slow down. We take cars instead of walking or biking. We stay home instead of going out to a gym or to play tennis.

And most of all, we watch too much television. With jobs that require more thought and less muscle, we are turning into a nation of couch potatoes. For many people, the most exerting activity in a day is pushing the buttons on the remote control. At least in years gone by, we had to get up and walk across the room to change the channel! Now, through the wonders of modern technology, we can sit in a chair all night long, only rising long enough to attend to personal needs. But all this progress has left us soft! We can't keep up. We are becoming a population of overweight adults who will acquire a variety of medical problems, including vein disorders.

You say you don't have time to exercise. After chasing the kids all day and attending to work and household responsibilities, there's just nothing left. We know, we've said the same thing. But researchers have found that next to smoking, a sedentary lifestyle is the most common cause of death and disease in this country.[6] It would help all of us to at least try. A little effort goes a long way.

Before jumping into any new and strenuous activity that you may no longer be in shape for, seek the advice of your physician. Most of us remember ourselves as teenagers: young, energetic, and invincible; unfortunately, our bodies live in the present and not in past memories. Make sure you can live through your exercise. Start out slow and work up to things. Trying to be a high-caliber athlete on day one will lead to pain, injuries, and frustration. Remember, these activities are supposed to be fun, not more work.

No matter what you decide to do, from videotapes to expensive gyms with personal trainers, a few basic rules apply to all:[6]

1. Stop when your body tells you. This is especially important if you feel chest pain or tightness.
2. Gradually work up to your desired goal.
3. Spend a few minutes warming up before really exerting yourself.
4. Similarly, spend a few minutes cooling down at the end of your activities. This is often a good time to do stretching.

If exercise and sports don't interest you, don't despair. Walking is an excellent activity that is good for your cardiovascular system as a whole, and your leg veins specifically. During walking, the calf muscles help squeeze the blood pooled in the tissues of your legs and in the veins, markedly helping blood return to the heart.

Real walking means more than a stroll to look at the scenery. It means walking fast enough to increase your heart rate. This can be accomplished with a brisk pace. With this effort you can burn the same number of calories as if you had jogged the same distance.[6] But even slow walking has been shown to produce some benefit.

Some nice things about walking are that you can do it anywhere, it's relatively cheap, and all you really need is some motivation and a good pair of walking shoes. An easy way to help incorporate more walking into your daily life with little or no effort is to park your car a little farther from your destinations than you normally would. If you gradually increase this distance, you will be surprised how much walking you can add to your day. Another simple step is to use the stairs more often than the elevator. Start simple go down the stairs. Then slowly start going up more flights of steps. With time you'll be able to cover lots more ground and feel much better while doing it.

Getting started exercising or walking is half the battle. Keeping yourself motivated to continue doing it is the other half. We all have used the excuses, "It takes too long, I don't have time for it," "It's boring," "I'm not seeing any results." In order to keep us on track, the authors of *The Arthritis Cure* have come up with several useful suggestions:[6]

1. Keep an exercise calendar where you will see it all the time. Consider your mirror or refrigerator. Put a mark on it each time you exercise. The simple act of seeing this calendar will help reinforce the need to exercise.

2. Try to find a partner. If someone is depending on you, you'll be less inclined to skip or forget it.

3. Buy new equipment. Whether its shoes or a treadmill, most of us are motivated to use it if we spent money on it. The same holds true for health and fitness club memberships. Just remember to spend within your means. The idea is to exercise, not just look good in your new workout outfit.

4. Keep your equipment where it is visible. Out of sight is out of mind. Although many of today's exercise machines can be folded up and slipped out of sight, that's exactly the wrong thing for most of us to do. Keep it in plain sight. You'll be much more likely to use it if you don't need to think about where you put it.

5. Pick a goal. Most of us are goal-oriented. If you train for an event, you are much more likely to work harder.

6. Don't put it off. Think about exercising in the morning. That way it's done. Even if your day becomes chaotic, your workout is complete. Similarly, on days when you just don't feel like exercising, consider doing just a little. It keeps you in the swing of things, and once you start, you may just see it all the way through.

PRACTICE GOOD FOOT AND LEG HYGIENE

Often overlooked and underrated, various foot conditions can lead to serious infections that may be threatening to limb or even life. This is especially true in diabetics with impaired sensation in their feet due to nerve damage. Even trivial injuries such as cuts, scrapes, punctures, and even ingrown toenails can become serious problems in the right setting. If you have dry or flaky skin, use a moisturizing cream to prevent cracks and sores from developing. Make it a habit to inspect your feet and legs once a month. Do it when you do your breast self-examination. Better yet, check your feet and legs once a day as a preventative measure. If there is a problem or question, consult your doctor right away. Finding a venous leg sore early, when it is small, makes treatment and healing much easier, often without a long and complicated course. A few minutes a day can go a long way to averting bigger problems. So stop ignoring your feet in general, without them life is far less pleasant and far more complicated. On that note...

WEAR GOOD SHOES

Proper fitting shoes help prevent trivial injuries and many of the problems discussed in the previous paragraph, and they support your feet better as well. Sometimes pain attributed to varicose veins and chronic venous insufficiency can be improved with good shoes. The placement of custom supports, known as orthotics, can often help. Good shoes will make you and your feet feel better. They may even help you avoid something more serious and extensive later on. The importance of good shoes cannot be overemphasized.

CONSIDER WEARING COMPRESSION STOCKINGS

Consider wearing 40 mm elastic compression stockings for most standing activities. The development of modern fabrics has made them more like fine fashion hosiery. Unattractive, uncomfortable, bulky elastic stockings are a thing of the past. It's a simple treatment that will clearly help your legs.

LEARN TO WALK PROPERLY

It has been found that improper alignment of body parts can lead to pain. As a result, health care providers who treat people in pain, such as sports medicine physicians, rheumatologists, osteopathic manipulators, physical therapists, and foot center physicians, have developed a significant interest in biomechanics, the study of how the body's movement exerts forces along muscles, bones, and joints. By teaching some patients the proper way to walk, and by placing patients in the proper shoes and supports, years of pain and suffering can be "cured" in a matter of weeks. Furthermore, by fixing problems at an earlier stage, long-term joint difficulties such as arthritis may be avoided. But seek help from a professional. Relieving leg pain may be just a correct step away.

AVOID INJURY

This may seem obvious, but many people overlook simple methods of preventing injuries. Probably the easiest way to prevent serious injuries is to wear your seat belt and shoulder strap. Unfortunately, even in this day and time, people still don't follow this simple recommendation. There is little doubt that these two measures have saved far more lives and prevented more injuries than they could have ever contributed to. By limiting injuries associated with major bone fractures and hospitalizations with prolonged recoveries, often involving long periods of bed rest, you decrease the likelihood you will develop a deep vein thrombosis and the associated life-threatening blood clot thrown to the lung.

Prevent sports-related injuries by getting in shape and staying that way. When a new sports season roles around, train appropriately to avoid hurting yourself. If you plan a snow-skiing trip in the winter, spend some time in the late fall stretching and building strength in the necessary muscle groups, while you continue your general workout as part of a balanced exercise program.

Wear the appropriate attire for each specific sport and activity. Proper shoes have been developed for all types of high-impact events. These will maximize results and minimize difficulties. If you're playing tennis, wear shoes made for this, jogging shoes for jogging, and so forth.

TRAVELING

When traveling long distances in an automobile, stop the car and get out and walk around every 1 or 2 hours. The same holds true on airplanes. Get up and walk in the aisles. If you have a layover, get out and walk in the terminal. Walking helps the calf muscle pump move the blood that was stagnant or flowing slowly in the veins during prolonged periods of sitting. Additionally, a recent study has documented that traveling more than 4 hours seems to increase the risk for deep vein thrombosis during the next month.[7] Any activity that decreases venous pooling may decrease thromboses.

Most hotels now have fitness clubs to keep you in step while away from home. You may have to modify your normal routine, but at least you're doing something. If no gym is available, consider aerobic exercises in your room or walking. If you are alone or don't feel safe walking outside, then consider walking around a secure area in the hotel.

DECREASE SUN EXPOSURE

When we were children, we all worshipped the sun. Many of us lay out in the sun for hours to get a bronze sun-tanned body. Hollywood and the magazines have portrayed beauty as having a tan. Furthermore, the jet-set crowd has always been shown on exotic beaches and resorts.

Pale, white skin was just not desirable. But now we're paying for it with our lines and wrinkles and the unfortunate dramatic rise in the incidence of melanoma, the most deadly of all the skin cancers. Now we're suffering. How does this relate to veins? It appears that significant sun exposure can be linked to the development of facial spider veins.

What can we do now? There is no better time to make lifestyle changes and try to decrease sun exposure. When outside always try to wear a large hat. Some countries such as New Zealand have already mandated this in the schools. Also try to wear sun block, 30 strength or stronger, to stop some of the harmful rays.

UNCROSS YOUR LEGS

Although no good data support the theory that leg crossing causes varicose veins, some information does indicate that it increases the pressure in your leg veins.[14] Since vein pressure increases while people sit in a chair, following the same logic, it only stands to reason that the same may hold true for crossing the legs.[8]

AVOID TIGHT-FITTING CLOTHING

Fashion styles come and go, but varicose veins are yours to keep. Although primarily a theoretical concern, tight-fitting clothes, such as boots that fit snugly against the back of the knee and jeans that are tight in the groin, may block venous return. One study has found a high incidence of varicose veins in women who wear corsets compared to those who wear looser attire.[15] Even though this clearly is not a cause-and-effect finding, over the years tight-fitting clothes may contribute to the development of varicosities in those prone to the problem.[8]

A FEW THOUGHTS ABOUT PREGNANCY

Women tend to be more prone to vein problems during pregnancy for three main reasons (discussed in the chapter dealing with varicose veins): hormonal changes, changes in the circulating blood volume, and increased pressure from the uterus on pelvic and leg veins. But in addition, as the months progress during pregnancy, many women become less and less active. This is easy to understand: The effects of the expanding uterus begin to take their toll. The future mother and her family also undergo dramatic lifestyle changes in preparation for the birth of a child.

Before doing anything drastic to counteract the stresses of pregnancy on your body, it's always best to seek the advice of your physician or nurse-midwife. They, more than anyone else, know what you should and shouldn't be doing. But unless you are on bed rest or have significant restrictions, some general recommendations may make your life more comfortable along the way. Also, keep it in mind that many vein problems resolve after delivery.

First, try to walk as much as possible to keep the calf muscle pumps functioning. If you are unable to walk or must stand in one place for a long time, tense the muscles in your calf, then roll up and down on the balls of your feet to help pump the blood along. This can be done when standing in line at the grocery store or when waiting for an elevator, even if you're not pregnant.

Next, elevate your legs whenever possible, but at least at some point every morning and afternoon, and preferably above the level of your heart. This activity will help drain any pooled blood and will counteract the gravitational effects of standing.

Also, start wearing prescription elastic compression stockings early in your pregnancy. You will probably need to ask your doctor about these; doctors rarely mention stockings since most people don't want to be bothered. But since you are reading this book, you're not like most people— you want to avoid the problem, not be stuck looking for ways to treat it. Special stockings that expand as your belly expands are required, so don't skimp on quality to get a cheaper price. If the stockings don't fit correctly, you won't wear them. You will be out the money without gaining any benefit. Always put them on first thing in the morning, wear them all day, take them off at night, then bathe and retire to bed. Putting them on after you have been standing for awhile allows more blood to pool in your legs. This makes the stockings tighter and harder to get on, which decreases their effectiveness and your willingness to wear them.

Recently, elastic harnesses that go on like a vest have been developed to help elevate your belly. These devices alleviate some back pain, but they may also help decrease pelvic venous congestion by lifting the uterus off the pelvic veins. As a result, there may be less leg vein obstruction as well.

One brief mention of a very common, oftentimes very painful, but seldom discussed problem: vulvar varicosities, similar to leg vein varicosities, develop in the inner thigh and labial region. They are similar to the development of rectal hemorrhoids during pregnancy, only less common. Special elastic stockings have been developed to compress the crotch region, which decreases the swelling of these uncomfortable varicosities. Fortunately for most women afflicted with this problem, they usually resolve after delivery.

CHAPTER 11

What's on the Horizon?

For years, vein problems have been left to the most junior physicians or those that were in the twilight of their careers. No one wanted to manage the never-ending sores or big swollen legs of patients with venous insufficiency. Vein surgery was never glamorous, and those who showed an interest in it were often criticized by their peers.

But times are changing! Vein centers with sincere interest in these problems are popping up throughout this country and the world. They dispense state-of-the-art techniques for treating even the most complex problems. Instead of seeing vein problems as a cosmetic nuisance, vein center staffs have a dedicated interest in seeing that these conditions are recognized for what they are: medical problems that require well-thought-out plans of action.

With new interest in this area, research and dollars for new treatment methods have come pouring in from both the private sector and universities, which helps to clarify proper treatment methods. We have reached only the tip of the iceberg in terms of treating vein problems in order to prevent further troublesome conditions.

PREVENTION

Clearly, prevention is the best approach to any health problem, and vein problems are no exception to the rule. Unfortunately, at this time, the most common blood vessel problems, spider veins and varicose veins, do not have well-defined causes. Methods for preventing problems such as venous stasis disease will be discussed in the following sections. More approaches to prevention are addressed in the chapter, "What You Can Do to Help Yourself."

GENE THERAPY

It is undeniable that heredity plays a large role in the development of varicose and spider veins. Up to 80% of the women in our practice report a parent or grandparent with varicose veins. In the case of spider veins most women report a sister, mother, or grandmother with this problem. Some studies report that 90% of vein patients have a positive family history of varicose or spider veins. Investigators have also found that mothers and daughters, as well as identical twins, often have spider veins in the same distribution on their legs.[1] Is this coincidence? Probably not.

Researchers have also shown that certain races have more of a tendency to varicose vein formation than the population as a whole. People of Irish descent have a higher incidence than those of Scottish or English heritage. African blacks have a much lower incidence than American blacks, whose rates are similar to that of American whites.[2] Although there are cultural and environmental differences in all these groups, the trends lead one to suspect heredity plays an important role.

With the intense focus on genetic code research, and with the ability pharmaceutical companies have to manipulate this information and develop better medications, we believe it is only a matter of time until a gene or genes associated with varicose and spider veins will be identified. Once that occurs, selective gene therapy will provide targeted treatment, possibly before a problem occurs. Presumably, gene therapy will allow site-specific alterations that will reverse or stop a problem. Although still well down the road, these findings will probably occur in our lifetime or our children's, causing a radical change in the way we treat these conditions. With this technology, however, will come ethical questions regarding what to do with this information and our newfound capabilities, similar to the recent discussions surrounding the cloning of a sheep. Fortunately, with vein conditions we are generally not dealing with life-and-death problems. The issues are the same, but there is an order of magnitude difference in the complexity of the solutions.

CREAMS, LOTIONS, AND TONICS

Touted through the centuries by traveling hucksters at circus side-shows, and now in the information age through magazine advertisements and television infomercials, to our knowledge not a single topical product has withstood the test of time in treating spider veins, facial veins, or varicose veins. Some people have reported promising initial results, but long-term follow-up has been lacking.

Studies are underway, however, to try and develop drug products to treat vein conditions that are similar to the patches and chewing gums that help people stop smoking, and the creams and now a pill to return hair to bald men. The pharmaceutical industry is looking into these problems with vigor. If only a portion of the greater than 80 million people in the United States sought treatment, the revenue would be staggering, let alone considering the dollars to be made world-wide. With the potential millions of affected consumers in this country, and at least a billion or more people worldwide, the revenue involved is mind boggling. We expect an effective cream for spider veins early in the twenty-first century that will completely revolutionize the treatment of vein problems.

One herb to watch in the future is horse chestnut seed extract. Some initial studies appear to look promising.

LASERS FOR SPIDER VEINS

Newer and better lasers will allow more rapid treatment of spider veins, a very common condition. Also, side effects will diminish as advances are made. Eventually, we suspect, single treatment sessions will become the mainstay for laser therapy. Also, as it was with computers, the cost of building and purchasing this equipment will decrease, and this savings can be passed on to the patient; then, treatment will be available to a greater number of people.

SCLEROTHERAPY FOR SPIDER VEINS

Long the mainstay of treatment for this problem, its place will most likely change to helping lasers rather than vice versa. Since the sclerosing solutions are quite good at this time, little research will occur in developing new formulas. Therefore, this treatment will stagnate as others take off.

SCLEROTHERAPY FOR VARICOSE VEINS

With the scientific data mounting that sclerotherapy should primarily be used on small varicose veins, acceptance by physicians of its proper role in treatment will follow.[3-8] This will allow for better long-term results and less complications from varicose vein treatment.

SURGERY FOR VARICOSE VEINS

As more and more information is gained about the role of varicose vein problems in leading to chronic venous insufficiency and open sores, we believe surgery will play a bigger role in prevention and treatment. Minimally invasive techniques and their widespread use by the surgical community will return surgical procedures to their proper place in treating vein problems. The well-deserved bad name given to the classical vein stripping operation and its painful long-term recovery will be replaced with a host of new techniques. Office surgery, even on the most extensively diseased legs, allows for substantial cost savings and minimal discomfort. People are able to return to work and their normal activities more rapidly. Individuals will seek treatment at an earlier stage and will endure fewer years of suffering, discomfort, and unfortunate long-term effects on their legs and bodies as a whole.

ELASTIC COMPRESSION THERAPY

Similar to some of the findings discussed with varicose vein surgery, long-term compression is better than no therapy at all for minor varicosities and for those too ill to be treated or who refuse treatment. The issue of the chronically swollen leg in chronic venous insufficiency is well known. The more swollen the leg, the more problems are encountered. By placing people in compression stockings, the problems associated with these conditions can be decreased.

For years many physicians, including the authors, have tried to encourage people to wear compression stockings, but this view has not been universal. Now, using compression stockings for long-term treatment of patients who have suffered a lower extremity blood clot or have venous insufficiency is gaining widespread acceptance. If all doctors would uniformly place people with these problems in hose, many of the late and chronic problems such as open sores will be decreased or avoided.

With the development of new thinner materials, and with a variety of colors and styles, patients should be more willing to wear hose. They no longer look like your grandmothers old thick leggings. They are now virtually indistinguishable from everyday fine fashion hosiery. The uncomfortable bulky material has been replaced with a silky, virtually transparent texture, and it is difficult if not impossible for others to know you are wearing them. This change in and of itself should lead to more women agreeing to wear the compression stockings over the long term.

BLOOD CLOTS IN THE LEGS

New, very accurate blood tests are being developed to help rapidly diagnose deep vein clots. These tests can give answers in the office or emergency room, avoiding costly and time-consuming ultrasounds and x-ray tests.[9,10]

An aggressive approach to the prevention of lower extremity blood clots is now underway by most physicians for hospitalized patients. Previously, patients at prolonged bed rest were only placed in very low compression stockings to prevent blood clots. Although the research data have shown that these are of benefit in preventing deep vein thromboses, they are not as effective in preventing leg swelling when the patient returns to walking. Many up-to-date doctors are now also looking to other methods of stopping blood clot formation.

In nonsurgical patients, the simple act of getting people up and out of bed several times a day has been found to be very useful. Placing a board at the foot of the bed so that people can push on it for exercise allows the calf muscle pumps to help force stagnant, slow-flowing, potentially clot-forming blood back into the system.

People known to have a high risk for developing blood clots, such as those who have previously had them or those with cancer, can be treated with many different approaches as a precaution. Blood-thinning medicines can run the gamut from the minimal effects of aspirin, which is recognized to work effectively preventing heart attacks and strokes but may do little for vein problems, to the full-blown effects of warfarin. In between, is a level where most people are treated.

Low-dose heparin, a modification of the medication injected into a vein, is commonly used as a clot-preventing drug. Usually given as shots twice a day under the skin, it is effective in preventing clot formation at minimal risk to the patient. This approach is gaining widespread enthusiasm in the medical community as there is a better understanding of the way blood clots develop. Furthermore, few complications leaves little downside and possibly a strong upside to using this drug routinely.

In the postsurgical patient, the use of blood thinners, even in low doses, is more of a problem. With low-dose heparin, studies have reported a mild increase in surgical bleeding and blood clot formation in the wound, which increases the incidence of wound infections. As a result, other kinds of treatments are now being more commonly used.

Intermittent pneumatic compression stockings have been used with great success. These plastic-sleeve-like devices, which fit over your legs like pants, have been developed to mimic the action of the calf muscle pumping the blood. When attached to an air compressor, these garments squeeze and massage the blood from your foot to your thigh, moving pooled blood from the deep veins back to your heart. Since the construction of these devices has been refined, these stockings are not uncomfortable and are well tolerated by patients.

Once a blood clot has developed, aggressive management is needed to limit vein valve damage as much as possible. Some of the treatments have been touched on in the chapter on lower extremity blood clots. If the clot is found very early, very strong clot-dissolving medications can be given by catheters directly to the affected site. As the ability to perform these invasive procedures reaches more hospitals, we feel this approach to early deep vein thromboses will expand, leading to a decrease in the long-term problems of chronic venous insufficiency and swollen, sore-ridden legs.

Safer short- and long-term clot-dissolving agents are also being developed that will treat recent deep vein clots on an outpatient basis, instead of with hospitalization. It appears that these new medicines can be given once or twice a day by injection just below the skin rather than continuously through the vein.[11] This is similar to the way low-dose heparin is given to prevent clot formation. These new medications may be more cost-effective and clinically safer than the older drugs. Better blood test monitoring of these medications makes these drugs safer to use. This decreases the reluctance of physicians to place people on them for long periods of time. In fact, some of the newest and apparently safest medications don't even require blood test monitoring at all.

CHRONIC VENOUS INSUFFICIENCY

One of the most startling recent findings was that many patients with chronic venous insufficiency never had deep vein blood clots. In many cases, skin changes were not from longstanding deep vein obstruction. We now know that leaky vein valves rather than blockage are the main culprits in these findings.[12-16] In up to 20% of patients, untreated varicose veins may be the only cause for these terrible problems. Treatment of the varicose veins may then stablize or reverse some of the findings.

Researchers are now exploring the effectiveness of transplanting vein valves from a good leg to an injured one to help reestablish the integrity of the deep vein system, which lowers the venous pressure in the legs and decreases side effects. Cadaver veins and possibly synthetic materials may be used for this surgery. With the use of endoscopic techniques, direct repair of the injured valves may be possible in our lifetime.[17] This technique may be appropriate for a highly select group of patients.

Leg ulcers continue to be a treatment dilemma. Various creams and compounds have been tried, but in our opinion, good-old soap and water usually works just as well and is a lot cheaper. In certain instances, special ulcer healing kits may also be appropriate. For really bad, difficult-to-heal ulcers, surgeons have reluctantly recommended a very extensive operation in the past. Although ulcers often healed with this surgical method, frequent wound complications and long hospitalizations were the norm. A recent endoscopic approach to this procedure has markedly diminished the problems and moved it into an outpatient setting.[19] The data are limited but very promising for improved treatment of this very bad problem.

Researchers are also looking at hormones and growth factors that may speed up wound healing. Several studies show faster results compared to conventional therapies.[20] If these findings hold up in the long term, they will completely revolutionize the treatment of this difficult, recurring problem.

UPPER EXTREMITY BLOOD CLOTS

Understanding that upper extremity blood clots are a serious problem is a great advance. This condition is becoming more common each year as more and more catheters are placed in blood vessels for long-term treatments. Research is underway to investigate the way catheters are made so they can be coated with materials that block clot formation. This may lead to a decrease in the occurrence. Once a clot develops, aggressive management, often with rapid, powerful clot-dissolving medicine is required, if a usable arm is to result.

CHAPTER 12

Commonly Asked Questions

1. HOW DO I KNOW WHICH PROBLEM I HAVE?

Varicose veins, spider veins, and all of the other vein problems discussed in this book are true medical conditions. As with other medical problems, your physician can be the best source of information to help with the diagnosis and treatment of these disorders. Oftentimes you will be referred to a dermatologist, general surgeon, plastic surgeon, or vascular surgeon to assist in diagnosis or treatment; however, whenever there is a question regarding the problem at hand, seeing your doctor or a vein care specialist is the best way to obtain timely and current information. This book can also aid in helping you sort out one problem from another.

2. DOES THIS MEAN THAT I HAVE A CIRCULATION PROBLEM?

Physicians and the medical community generally regard a circulation problem as something related to the arteries that carry the blood away from the heart to the rest of your body. Atherosclerosis, or hardening of the arteries, is a good example of a circulation problem. This problem can affect the arteries of your heart, and when an artery in your heart becomes sufficiently blocked, a heart attack will ensue. Generally speaking, vein problems are not considered a "circulation" disorder.

3. WHAT ARE SPIDER VEINS?

Spider veins are small, slightly dilated veins that connect to the capillaries where oxygen is delivered to the tissues. They are located right under the skin surface and generally appear as tiny red or purple lines, which can also be in clusters. Frequently located on the thighs and calves, some people can have them on the face, especially around the nose. They serve no real purpose. Treatment produces no bad effects.

4. WHAT CAUSES SPIDER VEINS?

There is no good answer to this question. Heredity plays a major role. If your parents have them, there is a good chance you will as well. The other important risk factor is being female. Many researchers think that formation of these veins is influenced by the hormones estrogen and progesterone. Injuries to an area also can play a role. When these veins appear on the face, it is believed that longstanding sun exposure is the cause, but an absolute answer is still not available as to why they develop and in whom.

5. CAN I HAVE SYMPTOMS FROM MY SPIDER VEINS?

Many patients have no symptoms with their spider veins. But a large number of women experience pain, itching, and burning. The only way to get rid of these symptoms is to treat the spider veins.

6. WHAT ARE THE MOST COMMON TREATMENTS FOR SPIDER VEINS?

Worldwide, injection sclerotherapy is the number one treatment for spider veins. With the recent development of laser and laser-like pulsed-light systems, many patients are being treated without needles and injections.

7. WHAT ARE VARICOSE VEINS?

Varicose veins are blood vessels that have lost their normal shape, often because of abnormally functioning vein valves. Common causes include being born with fewer valves than is normal (the heredity effect) and injuries to the valves from blood clots. When the one-way valves start to leak, blood pools in the vein and its walls become distended. The vein then loses shape and becomes malformed and prominent. Generally these veins appear as bulging, abnormally enlarged, blue, rope-like veins found on the leg. Most varicose veins occur on the inner aspect of the thigh or calf, or in the back of the leg, knee, and calf. These distributions are consistent with the regions served by the greater saphenous and lesser saphenous veins, which make up the superficial vein system that drains the leg.

8. WHAT CAUSES VARICOSE VEINS?

As with spider veins, there is no definite answer to this question. We do know that heredity plays a significant role. Studies have found that when both parents had varicose veins, 85% of their children had evidence of varicosities as well. When only one parent was affected, only 41% of the children had varicose veins. When neither parent had varicose veins, only 27% of the children had them.[1] This data has been substantiated in another series that found only 28% of patients with varicose veins had a negative family history for them.[2] So when all other answers fail, we can always blame our parents for this problem. Some scientists also believe that they have recently identified a gene that causes varicose veins. Other factors may be obesity, prolonged sitting, and pregnancy. The female hormones estrogen and progesterone also seem to play a significant role in the development of varicose veins, which may explain why they are more prevalent in women than men.

9. WHAT ARE THE SYMPTOMS OF VARICOSE VEINS?

Patients commonly report a dull-aching, tired feeling in their legs when standing or sitting for prolonged periods of time. These symptoms seem to worsen as the day goes along. Some patients report isolated spots of tenderness along the rope-like bulging areas, especially in varicose veins along the outside aspect of the calf. Most people find relief with leg elevation; however, patients should seek evaluation by their physician to rule out other blood vessel disorders before blaming all leg pain on varicose veins.

10. WHAT ARE THE MOST COMMON TREATMENTS FOR VARICOSE VEINS?

The treatment should be tailored to the individual patient. Patients with minimal symptoms and findings may require minimal treatment. Patients with severe findings may require more aggressive treatment. Use of elastic compression stockings is the simplest course of action. Stockings will not cure varicose veins, but they will assist in supporting the vein wall and reconfiguring vein valves so they function more normally. They also prevent leg swelling. The key to using elastic stockings is to put them on as soon as you get out of bed in the morning and then keep them on all day. Elastic stockings require a careful fit and generally should be replaced every 4 to 6 months.

Injection sclerotherapy is not generally recommended for patients with large varicose veins, varicose veins extending up to the groin, or people who are significantly overweight. It can be used effectively for small (less than 3 mm) varicose veins or veins that remain after surgery. The recurrence rate after injection sclerotherapy in large varicose veins is quite high. Similarly, injections in the groin may lead to a leakage of the hardening solution into the deep veins, which might lead to a deep vein clot and its associated problems. Thus, although injection sclerotherapy can be quite useful in small varicose veins and spider veins, it is usually a poor method for treating large varicose veins. Surgery is the best treatment presently available for removing large varicose veins, and it can easily be performed in an office setting under local anesthesia. Only the damaged segments of the vein are removed through very small microsurgical incisions. The remaining normal veins are left intact. This leads to a very nice cosmetic and functional result.

11. SHOULD ALL VARICOSE VEINS BE TREATED?

The answer to this is yes and no. There are two main types of varicose veins. Primary varicose veins are those that you inherit from your parents, or develop with pregnancy, obesity, and so forth. These are the most common type of varicose veins. They can be treated by all of the previously described methods. Secondary varicose veins, however, occur after an injury to your leg or after the development of a deep vein clot.

These varicose veins may become responsible for carrying the bulk of the blood flow back to the heart when a blood clot or scarring obstructs the return of blood flow through the deep venous system. In this case, removal or sclerotherapy of these veins can lead to far worse problems than the varicose veins themselves. In this situation, compression stockings are the only recommended method of long-term treatment.

Another type of secondary varicose veins are those that sometimes recur following surgery or sclerotherapy. These veins may have been invisible prior to their treatment, but after therapy blood flows via a different path to the heart, and these veins may become more obvious. These secondary varicose veins can be treated like primary varicose veins. If they develop shortly after surgery or are small, then injection sclerotherapy is often the best treatment. If years have passed since they were first treated, and the veins are large, surgery may be the best option. Your doctor or a vein care specialist would best be able to recognize the various types of varicose vein problems and recommend the proper treatment in the proper setting.

12. WHAT ARE THE MOST COMMON COMPLICATIONS OF VARICOSE VEINS?

The most common complications that we see for varicose veins are pain, phlebitis (inflammation of the vein), and thrombophlebitis (inflammation with a clot in the vein). Recently, studies have shown that venous leg sores are often related to underlying varicose veins. Leg swelling can also be seen with varicose veins. Primarily however, most people with varicose veins complain of aching, tired legs.

13. HOW CAN I PREVENT VARICOSE VEINS?

This is a difficult task since most varicose veins are inherited or hormonally related. Certainly, you should find ways to ensure that you don't become overweight because the increased pressure on the veins in your legs due to obesity can lead to more rapid development of varicose veins. Also, if you are sitting or standing for long periods of time, try to walk around. On long car trips, this should be done every

1 or 2 hours. This will improve the functioning of the vein muscle pump that helps blood return to your heart. Early use of compression stockings may also slow development.

14. HOW DO I TELL ONE LEG PAIN FROM ANOTHER?

Your doctor is the best person to answer this question. Certain patterns of pain are associated with certain problems. Pain related to varicose veins is most often described as an aching, tired sensation in your legs. Frequently this improves with walking as the muscle pump forces blood to return to your heart. This is different from the pain found in artery blockages, described as claudication, which worsens with walking and is only relieved with rest. At very late stages of arterial blockage, a phenomenon known as "rest pain" develops where severe pain occurs in the forefoot while lying in bed. Further elevation of the leg on pillows only makes the rest pain worse. The pain can be resolved only by hanging the leg over the side of the bed or trying to get up and walk. This is a very late finding. This problem leads to limb loss. The best way to sort out leg pain is to see your doctor. (Table I)

TABLE 1
Symptoms of Artery and Vein Problems

	ARTERIAL	VENOUS
Pulses	Decreased or absent	Normal, though they may be difficult to feel through swollen and thickened skin.
Color	Pale, especially on elevation; dark red on dependency.	Normal to blue color on dependency.
Pain	Develops in the muscles of the calf, thigh, or buttock with walking; resolves with rest.	Dull ache that usually improves with walking, elevation, or use of compression stockings.
Temperature	Cool.	Normal or warm.
Swelling	Absent.	Present, sometimes severe.
Skin changes	Thin, shiny skin; loss of hair over calves, feet and toes; thickened nails.	Brown colored; thickened skin, often with dermatitis.
Ulcer	Often involves toes or pressure areas on feet.	Usually develops near sides of ankles.

15. CAN VARICOSE VEINS COME BACK AFTER TREATMENT?

If elastic compression stockings are used as a primary treatment method for varicose veins, then certainly when you take them off, varicose veins will reappear. The compression stockings improve the symptoms, but do not treat the underlying vein abnormalities. With compression stockings the faulty veins have never been removed or treated, only the symptoms have been alleviated.

Injection sclerotherapy of large varicose veins has also not produced good long-term results. In a recent study, recurrence rates of 100% were documented one year after injection sclerotherapy.[3] After surgery there is no recurrence of the treated veins because they are no longer present. Occasionally a few missed veins, or more commonly new veins, can be identified as the blood finds alternate paths back to the heart. These new varicosities can be treated with any of the previously described methods.

16. WHY DO WOMEN GET MORE VARICOSE VEINS THAN MEN?

Varicose veins are common in both men and women. More than 50% of adult men and 66% of adult women are afflicted with this disorder.[4] The absolute reason why women develop more varicose veins than men has not been found, but it seems to be related to the female sex hormones estrogen and progesterone. Women are particularly vulnerable during the two times these hormones are most in flux: pregnancy and menopause. Oral contraceptives, better known as birth control pills, and hormone replacement therapy with estrogen and progesterone seem to also increase the likelihood of developing varicose veins. Some studies have implicated estrogen and others progesterone as the culprit.

Apparently, varying levels of estrogen and progesterone in the bloodstream change the structure and strength of the vein walls. In addition, the circulating blood volume that the veins must hold increases at times during a woman's life. During the menstrual cycle there is an increase of blood flow, and there is approximately a 150% increase in blood flow for pregnant women. Also during pregnancy the veins in the abdomen, pelvis, and legs are under much greater pressure due to the growth of the baby in the uterus. This appears to be why many pregnant women develop varicose veins.

17. DOES SMOKING PLAY A ROLE IN VARICOSE VEIN DEVELOPMENT?

It has not been shown that smoking directly causes varicose veins, but this connection has not been investigated in any significant detail. It is well established that other blood vessel problems such as heart disease are strongly linked to the use of cigarettes, so it only stands to reason that this link will be demonstrated for varicose veins as well. It has however been shown that the blood clots in the deep and superficial leg veins substantially increase when a woman on birth control pills also smokes.

18. WHAT IS PHLEBITIS?

The definition of phlebitis is "an inflammation of the lining of the vein." On examination there is a swollen, red, and tender area overlying the involved vein that may develop into thrombophlebitis, where a blood clot forms in the vein as well. These problems are frequently seen with varicose veins. With these conditions, similar symptoms may be present such as an area of swelling and a warm place tender to the touch. A dull aching feeling in the leg may be present. Oftentimes a hard, cord-like area can be felt in the vein when a clot develops. Both of these problems are generally treated with warm compresses, anti-inflammatory agents (like aspirin), and compression stockings. Patients should be encouraged to walk in an effort to stop further pooling of blood in the veins. This decreases the chance the clot will get larger. Going to bed for a week with your leg up is absolutely the wrong thing to do.

19. WHAT IS A DEEP VEIN THROMBOSIS?

Blood clots or "thrombi" that develop in the deep veins of the legs, close to the bone, are called deep vein thromboses. They are frequently associated with prolonged bed rest, trauma, and surgical procedures associated with bed rest, malignancy, and infection, but they are not directly associated with varicose veins. Deep vein thrombosis is a very serious, life-threatening problem, especially in the worst-case scenario where blood clots are thrown to the lungs, which can cause rapid death. The most common treatment for deep vein thrombosis is anticoagulation, both short and long term. All patients should be placed in compression stockings in an effort to decrease the severity of the subsequent chronic venous insufficiency, which can often lead to years of pain and suffering.

20. WHAT IS A PULMONARY EMBOLISM?

A pulmonary embolism is a blood clot that breaks loose from a vein in another location, travels through the bloodstream, through the right side of the heart, and then lodges in the blood vessel to the lung. When it does, that area of the lung can no longer transfer oxygen to the blood. Estimates are that 90% of the blood clots have come from the leg.[5] Approximately 650,000 cases of pulmonary embolism occur in the United States each year; up to 30% of these result in death.[5]

21. WHAT IS CHRONIC VENOUS INSUFFICIENCY?

Chronic venous insufficiency is decreased blood return from your legs. This clinical picture is usually the result of a deep vein blood clot, leaky valves, or varicose vein problems. Generally there is swelling and skin changes including an increase in skin pigmentation from light to dark brown. The legs also feel tired and heavy. As this problem progresses, sores can develop that have a tendency to repeatedly heal and break open.

This problem is very common. It has been suggested that chronic venous insufficiency affects nearly 20% of working men and women.[4] Approximately 10% of these individuals require hospitalization for a complication related to the problem.[6]

22. HOW DO I KNOW WHAT KIND OF LEG SORE I HAVE?

Once again, asking your physician is the best way to sort out the different problems that can be associated with leg ulcers. Many elderly patients have a venous leg ulcer. Some have too little arterial blood flow to the leg to allow for healing. To heal the leg ulcer, these patients may require intervention that will increase the blood flow. Some patients may think that an ulcer is venous, only to find it is related to trauma, an insect bite, or rarely, a cancer. Only with adequate evaluation by a properly trained physician can these problems be sorted out.

23. WHAT IS INJECTION SCLEROTHERAPY?

Injection sclerotherapy is a technique where a "hardening" agent is injected into spider veins so that a scar will develop. The solution causes the vein walls to become inflamed, and they seal themselves together. When veins can no longer carry blood, they are no longer visible through the skin. Certain veins require at least 4 treatments, possibly more, before they completely disappear.

24. WHAT IS A LASER?

Laser is an acronym for "*l*ight *a*mplification by *s*timulated *e*mission of *r*adiation." Basically, it is an intense burst of light that can cause a heat injury to tissues. Spider vein lasers destroy the tiny blood vessels. In recent years, lasers have had widespread use throughout all areas of medicine as both a diagnostic and a therapeutic tool.

25. WHAT CAUSES FACIAL SPIDER VEINS AND HOW DO YOU TREAT THEM?

Facial spider veins are similar to those found on the legs. They are often red in color. Blue veins are less common. They are probably the result of damaging effects of chronic sun exposure. The most common treatments involve lasers, electrosurgery, pulsed-light therapy, and to a limited extent, injection sclerotherapy.

26. HOW DOES BLOOD-THINNING MEDICINE WORK?

Blood-thinning medicine comes in two varieties. Heparin is administered through a vein, but it can also be injected into the fat on your belly. It is effective in minutes and lasts for several hours.

Warfarin is a pill. It works by interfering with blood-clotting factors dependent on vitamin K. Because it works indirectly, it takes several days to work and the effect lasts weeks when you stop taking it.

27. WHAT IS THROMBOLYTIC THERAPY?

Thrombolytic agents are very strong clot-dissolving medicines. They have specific indications in the treatment of blood clots and are usually given by a catheter directly into the clot. Unlike heparin and warfarin, they cannot be used for long periods of time as significant bleeding will result.

APPENDIX I

Societies that Can Provide Information about Physicians
in Your Area that Specialize in Vein Disorders

The American Venous Forum
13 Elm Street,
Manchester, MA 01944
Tel: (978) 526-8330
Fax: (978) 526-4018
www.venous-info.com

The British Venous Forum
The Royal Society of Medicine
1 Wimpole Street
London W1M 8AE
England

American College of Phlebology
100 Webster St.
Suite 101
Oakland, CA 94607
Tel: (510) 834-6500
Fax: (510) 832-7300
www.phlebology.org
e-mail: acp@amsinc.org
Your Local County Medical Society

Brochures

1. Treatment of leg veins
This brochure provides information about sclerotherapy and surgical
treatments for varicose veins. It was developed under the direction of
the board of directors of the North American Society of Phlebology.
Source:
North American Society of Phlebology
930 N. Meacham Rd.
Schaumberg, IL 60168-4014

2. Facts for consumers: Varicose vein treatments (#F030421)
This brochure was prepared with the assistance of the board of
directors of the American Venous Forum.
Source:
Federal Trade Commission
Bureau of Consumer Protection
Office of Consumer and Business Education
Washington, D.C. 20580

3. Sclerotherapy: Treatment of leg veins
This brochure describes the treatment of spider veins. There are no
color photographs of actual patients, but two-color diagrams of veins
and sclerotherapy treatment are included.
Source:
Contemporary Communications
P.O. Box 71985
Marietta, GA 30007

4. Questions and answers about sclerotherapy for varicose veins
This simple brochure provided as a patient education service by the
manufacturers of Sotradecol provides answers to ten commonly asked
questions about sclerotherapy. It was prepared with assistance from
the board of directors of the North American Society of Phlebology.
Source:
Wyeth-Ayerst Laboratories
P.O. Box 8299
Philadelphia, PA 19101

5. Spider vein, varicose vein therapy

This describes both varicose and telangiectatic leg veins (with a heavy concentration on "spider veins"). Operative and before-and-after color photographs are reproduced with excellent quality. The common patient questions are addressed and the common side effects of sclerotherapy are described.

Source:

American Academy of Dermatology

930 N. Meacham Rd.

P.O. Box 4014

Schaumberg, IL 60168-4014

6. Varicose veins

This information is provided by the United States National Heart, Lung and Blood Institute Information Center. It is a compilation of several easy-to-understand articles from the medical literature that provide an overview.

Source:

NHLBI Information Center

P.O. Box 30105

Bethesda, MD 20824-1015

(301) 251-1222

7. Varicose veins treatments (#327c)

This brochure was developed for the Consumer Information Center.

Source:

Consumer Information Center 6C

P.O. Box 100

Pueblo, CO 81002

8. The vein center brochure

This brochure was developed by our practice and is provided for general information purposes.

WELCOME

Approximately 80 million people in the United States suffer from varicose and spider veins. Some major causes of these conditions are heredity, prolonged standing, pregnancy, obesity, and aging. Even when spider and varicose vein problems do not cause pain and discomfort, many people seek treatment for cosmetic reasons. Whether medical or cosmetic, vein treatment can be rejuvenating.

The Vein Center offers a complete treatment program designed to meet your individual needs. You will receive modern and cosmetically superior treatment using the most advanced technology available. Under the direction of board-certified surgeons, our highly skilled physicians and staff work together to monitor your progress throughout the treatment process. They will ensure that the service you receive meets your individual needs.

Symptoms

Significant vein disease occurs in 3 out of 4 American women and 1 out of 5 American men. People with varicose veins may notice that their legs feel tired or heavy. They may experience pain, swelling, leg cramps, itching, or burning. Leg cramps often occur at night. Itching or burning usually occurs in areas of pigmentation or darkening of the skin. People with advanced stages of venous disease may develop phlebitis (an inflammation of the vein wall), dermatitis (inflammation of the skin over prominent varicose veins), or finally an ulceration (an open sore in the affected area).

COMMON VEIN DISORDERS

Varicose Veins

Varicose veins are abnormally enlarged veins, usually found on the legs. Blue rope-like veins occur when valves in connector veins malfunction. Smaller veins, close to the skin, swell and dilate when blood backs into them from larger, deeper veins. As a consequence of these changes, these veins lose their normal ability to carry blood back to the heart. Other veins in the leg then carry the blood originally carried by the malfunctioning veins.

Spider Veins

Spider veins, or telangiectasias, are bluish-red, web-like veins that commonly develop on the legs. These may occur on either leg alone or on both legs simultaneously, and may appear in clusters or as isolated threads. A larger underlying vein, usually not readily visible, often contributes to the development of spider veins. In some cases, clearing an area of spider veins may also require treating the larger vein. Spider veins have no real function.

TREATMENT METHODS

The Vein Center physicians and staff evaluate each patient individually to develop an appropriate and effective custom treatment plan. One or more of the following treatment methods may be used:

Pulsed-Light Therapy
    PhotoDerm VL™
Sclerotherapy
Microsurgical Therapy
    Scratching
    Ligation / Phlebectomy
Compression Stockings

PhotoDerm VL™

PhotoDerm VL™ is state-of-the-art technology using non-

invasive light therapy to eliminate small varicose and spider veins without injections or surgery. PhotoDerm VL™ uses intense, laser-like, pulsed light. It selectively penetrates the abnormal veins without damaging the surrounding tissue. A sequence of carefully calculated pulses cause the treated vein to clot and break down. These broken-down veins are absorbed by the body. Other existing blood vessels carry blood from the affected area back to the heart.

Treatment is applied by placing a handheld unit on your skin. Since PhotoDerm VL™ uses light rather than needles or incisions, treatment feels like a pinch or the snap of a rubber band. Local anesthetic or pain medication is not required.

This advanced technology effectively corrects spider veins and varicose veins of smaller diameters. Usually several treatments are required depending on the severity and density of the veins. Each session generally lasts twenty minutes. Your physician, considering the size and depth of your leg veins, will customize the treatment specifically for your skin type. You can return to work the same day and resume all regular activities. You should, however, limit exposure to the sun and high-impact aerobics for several days.

Some possible side effects of this treatment include a slight reddening of the skin or a local swelling that fades away within a few days. Occasionally, blistering or hypopigmentation, a lightening of the skin in the area where the PhotoDerm VL™ is applied, may occur. This may be avoided by staying out of the sun and advising the physician of any medications you are taking that may cause this photosensitivity. This is temporary and the skin will regain its normal color.

Sclerotherapy

Sclerotherapy is a widely used treatment method. The physician or nurse uses tiny needles to inject sclerosing (hardening) agents into an abnormal vein. The solution causes the interior of the vein to become scarred, which prompts the vein to close down. The body absorbs the scarred vein in the same way it absorbs a bruise. Blood flow remains unobstructed within other vessels in the area.

Some patients experience a mild burning sensation while the sclerosing agent enters the vein. However, most patients are pleasantly surprised at the minimal discomfort during treatment. Following treatment, there may be bruising for approximately 1 week. This bruising generally fades over a period of 3 to 4 weeks. Your physician will determine the appropriate amount of time between scheduled treatments and will also determine the number of treatments you will need to achieve maximum results. Following sclerotherapy, elastic compression stocking or ace wraps are worn for a specified period of time.

Scratching

This is a microsurgical technique that may be used for spider veins that are very close together. It effectively and very rapidly eliminates spider veins, requiring only a small incision approximately 1 mm in length. Unfortunately, most spider veins are not close together but are spread out, necessitating the use of injection sclerotherapy or pulsed-light therapy with the PhotoDerm VL™.

Ligation and Phlebectomy

Varicose veins that are large and protruding may require advanced testing to determine whether a major blood valve is functioning improperly. This is why some examinations with doppler ultrasound are done before initiating any procedure. Doppler also allows the physician to determine the exact flow of reflux blood in the vein and helps determine where the relatively painless microsurgical incisions will be placed. The varicose veins are then removed through very, very small incisions. In general, you may resume normal activities within 2 days of the procedure. Following vein surgery, elastic compression stockings are worn for a specified period of time.

We assure you that this procedure is relatively painless. It is safely done in our center without the need for hospitalization. It is a rather simple, yet very effective way to permanently remove unsightly varicose veins. We strive to attain the best cosmetic results possible, with a minimal amount of discomfort.

Compression Stockings

The mechanism by which fitted elastic compression stockings benefit patients with symptomatic venous disease is theoretical. It is believed that the bulging veins lying unsupported under the skin are compressed, lending support to their walls. This prevents the pooling of blood within these veins. The stockings also help control leg swelling, probably by forcing edema fluid back into the veins as the tissues under the skin are compressed.

The fit of these stockings is extremely important. Since elastic stretches, the stockings should be replaced every six months. The over-the-counter, off-the-shelf stockings labeled as beneficial for whatever ails one's legs probably have little merit and are not a good substitute for elastic compression stockings. Benefits derived from these over-the-counter stockings appear to be only subjective.

Recurrence

Patients who have a tendency to develop spider veins or varicose veins will most likely develop new veins during the course of their lifetime, regardless of the treatment modality used. The destroyed vessels will not return, but new veins may appear. For this reason, maintenance treatments of your legs may be necessary. The best time to treat new bothersome veins is when they are sufficiently developed to be clearly evident, but before they become extensive. Please feel free to discuss a vein maintenance schedule with our staff if this is something you feel might interest you.

Informational Web Sites

www.theveincenter.com
The Vein Center
Memphis, Tennessee
Bridget F. Ostrow, M.D.
Louis B. Ostrow, M.D.

* * *

www.veincenters.com
Midwest Vein Treatment Clinic, Inc.
Cincinnati Vein Center
Ronald G. Bush, M.D.
Lima, Dayton, and Cincinnati, Ohio
* * *
www.veinsonline.com

APPENDIX 2

Laser and Pulsed-Light Manufacturers
Unites States Offices
The following companies responded to
our request for corporate information:
Please contact these companies directly for a center near you.

Coherent Medical Group
2400 Condensa Street
Santa Clara, CA 95051
Tel: 800-227-1914 & 408-764-3000
Fax: 408-764-3999
Makers of: UltraPulse®-for laser skin resurfacing (CO_2)
UltraFine-for laser skin resurfacing (Erbium)
VersaPulse®-for vascular and pigmented lesions and tattoo removal
(multiple wavelengths)
LightSheer-for hair removal (diode system)

ESC Medical Systems Inc.
First Needham Place
250 First Avenue
Needham, MA 02194
Tel: 888-372-1001
Fax: 781-444-8812
www.escmed.com
Makers of: ESC Medical Systems manufacturers and
markets a variety of intense pulsed-light and laser products.
ESC offers full-featured systems for hair removal,
cellulite therapy, and other medical laser applications.
Products include Epilight System, EpiTouch Alexandrite and
Ruby Lasers for hair removal; PhotoDerm®VL/PL for benign
vascular and pigmented lesions/ PhotoDerm MultiLight for
large and deep benign vascular lesions, Derma K Dual-Wave CO_2/
Erbium Laser, NovaPulse® CO_2 Laser, and Silklaser Erbium
and CO_2 Lasers for resurfacing procedures; SilkLight Cellulite
Therapy, and a complete line of lasers for hospital
and office-based medical applications.

APPENDIX 3

Compression Stocking Companies
United States Offices
The following companies responded to
our request for corporate information:
Please contact them directly to get information on their
nearest supplier of stockings.

Beiersdorf-Jobst, Inc.
Box 471048
Charlotte, NC 28247-1048
Tel: 704-554-9933, 800-537-1063
Fax: 419-691-4511
Website: beiersdorf.com
Company contact: Marketing Communications
Makers of: Jobst Ultrasheer, Jobst for Men, Fast-Fit, Relief, Vairox
(All gradient compression hosiery)

Carolon
P.O. Box 1329
601 Forum Parkway
Rural Hall, NC 27045
Tel: 800-334-0414 & 336-969-6001
Fax: 336-969-6999
Website: www.carolon.com
E-mail address: carolon@carolon.com
Company contact: Scott Wilson
Makers of: "HealthSupport" compression hosiery
20-30mmHg, 30-40mmHg, 40-50mmHg

Coloplast Corporation
1955 West Oak Circle
Marietta, GA 30062-2249
Tel: 800-533-0464
Fax: 800-281-8504
Website: www.coloplast.com
Company contact: Liz Buffington, 800-788-0293, ext. 8445
Makers of: CircAid® Compression systems. It is a registered trade-
mark of CircAid Medical Products, Inc., San Diego, CA, USA, as are
the CircAid Theraboot and CircPlus™ appliances. These systems of
adjustable, non-elastic, nylon bands with Velcro® fasteners give the
patient the ability to sustain compression regardless of changes in
limb size, physical activity or underlying medical conditions.

Freeman Manufacturing Co.
900 W. Chicago Road
Sturgis, Michigan 49091-9756
Tel: 800-253-2091
Fax: 800-894-8248
Website: www.freemanmfg.com
E-mail address: freeman@freemanmfg.com
Company contact: Customer Service
Makers of: VENO-FLO™, Simply Support™,
Fashion Plus™ and Legato™.
Distributors of: Medi® and Jobst®

Julius Zorn, Inc. (JuZo)
P.O. Box 1088
Cuyahoga Falls, OH 44223
Tel: 888-255-1300
Fax: 330-916-9165
Website: http://www.juzousa.com
E-mail address: support@juzousa.com
Makers of: Support Hosiery, Support Socks,
Compression Stockings, Compression Arm Sleeves,
Hand Portions, Stump Shrinkers, Suspension Sleeves,
Knee Braces and Ankle Braces.

medi USA
76 West Seegers Road
Arlington Heights, IL 60005
Tel: 800-633-6334 & 847-640-8400
Fax: 847-640-0209
Website: www.mediusa.com
Company contact: Trish Herzog, Annie Silet
Makers of: Medi, the leader in medical compression stockings
for over 75 years, manufacturers each and every medi
medical stocking to meet the highest medical standards.
The result: uncompromising quality.

Sigvaris
1119 Highway 74
Peachtree City, GA 30269
Tel: 800-322-7744 & 770-631-1778
Fax: 800-481-5488 & 770-631-4883

REFERENCES

Introduction

1. MP Goldman, *Sclerotherapy Treatment of Varicose and Telangiectatic Leg Veins* (St. Louis, Missouri: Mosby, 1995), ix.

2. HC Baron and BA Ross, *Varicose Veins: A Guide to Prevention and Treatment* (New York: Facts on File, Inc. 1995), 33.

3. WW Coon, PW Willis III, and JB Keller, Venous Thromboembolism and Other Venous Disease in the Tecumseh Community Health Study, *Circulation* 48 (1973): 839.

4. M Lake, GH Pratt, and IS Wright, Arteriosclerosis and Varicose Veins: Occupational Activities and Other Factors, *JAMA* 119 (1942): 696.

5. EAV Tianco, G Buendia-Teodosio, and NL Alberto, Survey of Skin Lesions in the Philipino Elderly, *Int J Dermatol* 31 (1992): 696.

6. HC Baron and BA Ross, *Varicose Veins: A Guide to Preventing and Treatment* (New York: Facts on File, Inc. 1995), vii.

7. P Glovicki and JST Yao, *Handbook of Venous Disorders* (New York: Chapman and Hall Medical, 1996), xv.

8. CO Netzer and G Rudofsky, *Practical Ambulatory Phlebology* (Garching near Munich, Germany: Verlag Medical Concept GmbH, 1991), 7.

9. HC Baron and BA Ross, *Varicose Veins: A Guide to Prevention and Treatment* (New York: Facts on File, Inc. 1995), 1.

10. G Goren, *Office Phlebology: A Practitioner's Guide* (Encino, CA: Nerog-Hill Desktop Publishing, 1995), 4.

11. NL Browse and KG Burnand, The Postphlebitic Syndrome: A New Look, in JJ Bergan and JST Yao, *Venous Problems* (Chicago: Yearbook, 1978).

12. C Chess and Q Chess, Cool Laser Optics Treatment of Large Telangiectasia of the Lower Extremities, *J Dermatol Surg Oncol* 19 (1993): 74.

13. JL Villivicencio, Excision of Varicose Veins, in CB Ernst and JC Stanley, *Current Therapy in Vascular Surgery*, 2nd ed (Philadelphia: B.C. Decker, Inc. 1991.), 967.

Chapter 1: Understanding Your Circulation

1. HC Baron and BA Ross, *Varicose Veins: A Guide to Prevention and Treatment* (New York: Facts on File, Inc. 1995), pg 1.

2. S Mellander, Operative Studies on the Adrenergic Neuro-hormonal Control of Resistance and Capacitance Blood Vessels in the Cat, *Acta Physiol Scand* 50 (1960): 5.

3. MP Goldman, *Sclerotherapy Treatment of Varicose and Telangiectatic Leg Veins* (St. Louis, Missouri: Mosby, 1995), 85.

4. RL Waterfield, The Effect of Posture on the Volume of the Leg, *J Physiol* 72 (1931): 121.

5. J Ludbrook and J Loughlin, Regulation of Volume in Postarteriolar Vessels of the Lower Limb, *Am Heart J* 67 (1964): 493.

6. RF Rushmer, Effects of Posture, in RF Rushmer, *Cardiovascular Dynamics* (Philadelphia, WB Saunders, 1976).

Chapter 2: You and Your Doctors

1. AM Rapoport and AM Sheftell, *Headache Relief for Women* (Boston: Little, Brown and Company, 1995), 49.

Chapter 3: Spider Veins

1. NM Wilson and NL Browse, Venous Disease, in DL Clement and JT Shepherd, *Vascular Diseases in the Lower Limbs* (St. Louis: Mosby Yearbook, 1993).

2. LK Widmer, Peripheral Venous Disorders, *Basle Study III* (Berne, Switzerland: Hans Huber, 1978).

3. JK Rivers, PC Frederiksen, and C Dibdin, A Prevalence Survey of Dermatoses in the Australian Neonate, *J Am Acad Dermatol* 23 (1990): 77.

4. DM Duffy, Small Vessel Sclerotherapy: An Overview, *Adv Dermatol* 3 (1988): 221.

5. N Sadick, Treatment of Varicose and Telangiectatic Leg Veins with Hypertonic Saline: A Comparitive Study of Heparin and Saline, *J Dermatol Surg Oncol* 16 (1990): 24.

6. MP Goldman, *Sclerotherapy Treatment of Varicose and Telangiectatic Leg Veins* (St. Louis, Mosby, 1996.), 120.

7. AH Jacobs and RG Walton, The Incidence of Birthmarks in the Neonate, *Pediatrics* 58 (1970): 218.

8. B Cosman, Clinical Experience in the Laser Therapy of Port-wine Stains, *Lasers Surg Med* 1 (1980): 133.

9. WB Bean, *Vascular Spiders and Related Lesions of the Skin* (Springfield, IL: Charles C. Thomas, 1958).

10. SM Goodrich and JE Wood, Peripheral Venous Distensibility and Velocity of Venous Blood Flow During Pregnancy or During Oral Contraceptive Therapy, *Am J Obstet Gynecol* 90 (1964): 740.

11. LT Davis and DM Duffy, Determination of Incidence and Risk Factors for Rost-Sclerotherapy Telangiectatic Matting of the Lower Extremity: A Retrospective Analysis, *J Dermatol Surg Oncol* 16 (1990): 327.

12. HF Dvorak, Tumors: Wounds That Do Not Heal: Similarities Between Tumor Stroma Generation and Wound Healing, *New Engl J Med* 26 (1986): 1650.

13. D Clarke, A Martinez, and RS Cox, Analysis of Cosmetic Results and Complications in Patients with Stage I and II Breast Cancer Treated by Biopsy and Irradiation, *Int J Radiat Oncol Biol Phys* 9 (1983): 1807.

14. H Goldschmidt and WK Sherwin, Reactions to Ionizing Radiation, *J Am Acad Dermatol* 20 (1989): 278.

15. MP Goldman, *Sclerotherapy Treatment of Varicose and Telangiectatic Leg Veins* (St. Louis: Mosby, 1996), 200.

16. PA Ouvry and A Davy, The Sclerotherapy of Telangiectasia, *Phlebologie* 35 (1982): 349.

17. MP Goldman, *Sclerotherapy Treatment of Varicose and Telangiectatic Leg Veins* (St. Louis: Mosby, 1996), 280.

18. MP Goldman, *Sclerotherapy Treatment of Varicose and Telangiectatic Leg Veins* (St. Louis: Mosby, 1996), 431.

19. MP Goldman, Lasers and Noncoherent Pulsed-Light Treatment of Leg Telangiectasias and Venules, in MP Goldman and JJ Bergan, *Ambulatory Treatment of Venous Disease* (St. Louis: Mosby, 1996), 89.

20. C Chess and Q Chess, Cool Laser Optics Treatment of Large Telangiectasia of the Lower Extremities, *J Dermatol Surg Oncol* 19 (1993): 74.

21. Candela Corporation, The Candela Dynamic Cooling Device (Wayland, MA: Candela Corporation, 1997).

22. MP Goldman and S Eckhouse, ESC Medical Systems, Ltd. PhotoDerm VL Cooperative Study Group. Photothermal Sclerosis of Leg Veins, *Dermatol Surg* 22 (1996): 323.

23. ESC Medical Systems Ltd, Effective Treatment of Deep and Large Vessels with Vasculite™, *PhotoDerm*® *Application Notes* (Needham, MA: ESC Medical Systems Ltd, vol 1, no 6, 1998).

24. RG Bush, personal communication, 14 September 1998.

Chapter 4: Varicose Veins

1. I Prerovsky, Disease of the Veins, internal communication, MHO-PA 10964: World Health Organization.

2. HC Baron and BA Ross, *Varicose Veins: A Guide To Prevention And Treatment* (New York: Facts on File, Inc. 1995), 26.

3. MP Goldman, *Sclerotherapy Treatment of Varicose and Telangiectatic Leg Veins* (St. Louis, Missouri: Mosby, 1995), 56.

4. MP Goldman, *Sclerotherapy Treatment of Varicose and Telangiectatic Leg Veins* (St. Louis, Missouri: Mosby, 1995), 85.

5. J Troisier, Le Bayon: Etude genetique des varices. *Ann de Med* (France) 41 (1937): 30.

6. H Niermann, *Zwillingsdermatologie* (Berlin: Springer-Verlag, 1964).

7. JM Weddell, Varicose Veins Pilot Study, 1966, *Br J Prev Soc Med* 23 (1969): 179.

8. N Angle and JJ Bergan, Varicose Veins: Chronic Venous Insufficiency, in WS Moore, *Vascular Surgery: A Comprehensive Review* (Philadelphia: WB Saunders Company, 1997), 800.

9. HC Baron and BA Ross, *Varicose Veins: A Guide To Prevention And Treatment* (New York: Facts on File, Inc. 1995), 69.

10. WG Fegan, R Lambe, and M Henry, Steroid Hormones and Varicose Veins, *Lancet* 1 (1967): 1070.

11. NS Sadick, Predisposing Factors of Varicose and Telangiectatic Leg Veins, *J Dermatol Surg Oncol* 18 (1992): 883.

12. J Ludbrook, Obesity and Varicose Veins, *Surg Gynecol Obstet* 118 (1964): 843.

13. JC Seidell, Fat Distribution of Overweight Persons in Relation to Morbidity and Subjective Health, *Int J Obes* 9 (1985): 363.

14. TL Cleave, *On the Causation of Varicose Veins and Their Prevention and Arrest by Natural Means*: Bristol, Wright and Sons, 1960).

15. E Guberan et al, Causative Factors of Varicose Veins: Myths and Facts, *Vasa* 2 (1973): 115.

16. LK Widmer, Peripheral Venous Disorders: Prevalence and Sociomedical Importance: Observations in 4529 Apparently Healthy Persons, *Basle Study III* (Berne, Switzerland: Huber, 1978.)

17. AM Stewart, JW Webb, and D Hewitt, Social Medicine Studies Based on Civilian Medical Board Records. II. Physical and Occupational Characteristics of Men with Varicose Conditions, *Br J Prev Med* 9 (1955): 26.

18. CJ Alexander, Chair-Sitting and Varicose Veins, *Lancet* 1 (1972): 822.

19. JM Stanhope, Varicose Veins in a Population of Lowland New Guinea, *Int J Epidemiol* 4 (1975): 221.

20. HC Baron and BA Ross, *Varicose Veins: A Guide To Prevention And Treatment* (New York: Facts on File, Inc. 1995), 53.

21. EA Husni and WA Williams, Superficial Thrombophlebitis of the Lower Limbs, *Surgery* 91 (1982): 70.

22. JO Jorgensen et al, The Incidence of Deep Venous Thrombosis in Patients with Superficial Thrombophlebitis of the Lower Limbs, *J Vasc Surg* 18 (1993): 70.

23. EA Edwards, Thrombophlebitis of Varicose Veins, *Gynecol Obstet* 60 (1938): 236.

24. HP Totten, Superficial Thrombophlebitis: Observations on Diagnosis and Treatment, *Geriatrics* 22 (1967): 151.

25. WW Coon, PW Willis III, and JB Keller, Venous Thromboembolism and Other Venous Disease in the Tecumseh Community Health Study, *Circulation* 48 (1973): 839.

26. MP Goldman, *Sclerotherapy Treatment of Varicose and Telangiectatic Leg Veins* (St. Louis, Missouri: Mosby, 1995), 69.

27. MP Goldman, *Sclerotherapy Treatment of Varicose and Telangiectatic Leg Veins* (St. Louis, Missouri: Mosby, 1995), 200.

28. CO Netzer and G Rudofsky, *Practical Ambulatory Phlebology* (Garching Near Munich, Germany: Verlag Medical Concept GmbH, 1991).

29. M Henry, Injection Sclerotherapy for Varicose Veins: A View from Ireland, in MP Goldman and JJ Bergan, *Ambulatory Treatment of Venous Disease: An Illustrative Guide* (St. Louis, Missouri: Mosby, 1996), 99.

30. MP Goldman, *Sclerotherapy Treatment of Varicose and Telangiectatic Leg Veins* (St. Louis, Missouri: Mosby, 1995), 350.

31. RJ Tazelaar and HAM Neumann, Macrosclerotherapy and Compression, in MP Goldman and JJ Bergan, *Ambulatory Treatment of Venous Disease: An Illustrative Guide* (St. Louis, Missouri: Mosby, 1996), 105.

32. MP Goldman and JJ Bergan, *Ambulatory Treatment of Venous Disease: An Illustrative Guide* (St. Louis, Missouri: Mosby, 1996).

33. MP Goldman, *Sclerotherapy Treatment of Varicose and Telangiectatic Leg Veins* (St. Louis, Missouri: Mosby, 1995).

34. G Fegan, *Varicose Veins* (London, William Heineman, 1967).

35. P Wallois, The Conditions Necessary to Achieve an Effective Sclerosant Treatment, *Phlebologie* 35 (1982): 337.

36. JG Sladen, Combined Treatment, Flush Ligation, and Compression Sclerotherapy for Large Varicose Veins and Perforators, in MP Goldman and JJ Bergan, *Ambulatory Treatment of Venous Disease: An Illustrative Guide* (St. Louis, Missouri: Mosby, 1996), 113.

37. RL Kistner et al, The Evolving Management of Varicose Veins, *Postgrad Med* 80 (1986): 51.

38. SAA Beresford et al, Varicose Veins: A Comparison of Surgery and Injection/Compression Sclerotherapy Five-Year Follow-Up, *Lancet* 1 (1978): 921.

39. K Biegeleisen and RD Nielsen, Failure of Angioscopically Guided Sclerotherapy to Permanently Obliterate Greater Saphenous Varicosity, *Phlebology* 9 (1994): 21.

40. JT Hobbs, Surgery and Sclerotherapy in the Treatment of Varicose Veins, *Arch Surg* 190 (1974): 793.

41. E Einarsson, B Eklof, and P Neglan, Sclerotherapy or Surgery as Treatment for Varicose Veins: A Prospective Randomized Study, *Phlebology* 8 (1993): 22.

42. CCR Bishop et al, Realtime Color Duplex Scanning after Sclerotherapy of the Greater Saphenous Vein, *J Vasc Surg* 14 (1991): 505.

43. A Gongolo et al, Il Sistema Duplex nel Follow-Up della Terapia Sclerosante della Vena Grande Saphena, *Radiol Med* (Italy) 81 (1991): 303.

44. RM Knight, F Vin, and JA Zygmunt, Ultrasonic Guidance of Injections into the Superficial Venous System, Abstract 4S 14:50, presented at the 10th World Congress of Phlebology, Strasbourg, 2529 September 1989.

45. PK Thibault and WA Lewis, Recurrent Varicose Veins: Injection of Incompetent Perforating Veins Using Ultrasound Guidance, *J Dermatol Surg Oncol* 18 (1992): 895.

46. V Frederic and M Schadeck, Macrosclerotherapy and Duplex Technology, in MP Goldman and JJ Bergan, *Ambulatory Treatment of Venous Disease: An Illustrative Guide* (St. Louis, Missouri: Mosby, 1996), 141.

47. G Goren, *Office Phlebology: A Practitioner's Guide,* addendum vol (Encino, CA: Nerog-Hill Desktop Publishing, 1995), 41.

48. P Raymond-Martimbeau, Advanced Sclerotherapy Treatment of Varicose Veins with Duplex Ultrasonographic Guidance, *Semin Dermatol* 12 (1993): 123.

49. PK Thibault and WA Loweis, Recurrent Varicose Veins: Part 2: Injection of Incompetant Perforating Veins Using Ultrasound Guidance, *J Dermatol Surg Oncol* 18 (1992): 895.

50. V Frederick and M Schadek, Macrosclerotherapy and Duplex Technology, in MP Goldman and JJ Bergan, *Ambulatory Treatment of Venous Disease: An Illustrative Guide* (St. Louis, Missouri: Mosby, 1996), 141.

51. JJ Bergan, Clinical Application of Duplex Testing in the Treatment of Primary Venous Stasis, Varicose Veins, in PS Bemmelen and JJ Bergan, *Quantitative Measurement of Venous Incompetence* (Austin: RG Landes, 1992), 85.

52. G Goren, Injection Sclerotherapy for Varicose Veins: History and Effectiveness, *Phlebology* 6 (1991): 7.

53 JL Villanvicencio et al, Sclerotherapy for Varicose Veins: Practice Guidelines and Sclerotherapy procedures, in P Glovicki and JST Yao, *Handbook of Venous Disorders* (New York, 1996, Chapman and Hall Medical), 337.

54. W Benton, *Hippocratic Writings on Ulcers* (Chicago, Brittanica Great Books, 1970).

55. MP Goldman, *Sclerotherapy Treatment of Varicose and Telangiectatic Leg Veins* (St. Louis, Missouri: Mosby, 1995), 2.

56. H Kamal, *Encylcopedia of Islamic Medicine* (Cairo: General Egyptian Bood Organization, 1975), 724.

57. H Dodd and FB Cockett, *Pathology and Surgery of the Veins of the Lower Limbs* (Edinburgh: E&S Livingstone, Ltd.), 1956.

58. JJ Bergan, Ambulatory Surgery of Varicose Veins, in MP Goldman and JJ Bergan, *Ambulatory Treatment of Venous Disease: An Illustrative Guide* (St. Louis, Missouri: Mosby, 1996), 149.

59. DJ Tibbs, *Varicose Veins and Related Disorders* (Oxford: Butterworth/Heinemann, 1992), 377.

60. CV Ruckley, *Surgery for Varicose Veins* (London: Wolf Medical Publications, Ltd. 1983), 6.

61. S Ricci, M Georgiev, MP Goldman, *Ambulatory Phlebectomy: A Practical Guide For Treating Varicose Veins* (St. Louis, Missouri: Mosby 1995).

62. S Rivlin, The Surgical Cure of Primary Varicose Veins, *Br J Surg* 62 (1975): 913.

63. R Bush, Personal communication. 11 September 1998.

64. G Goren and AE Yellin, Minimally Invasive Surgery for Primary Varicose Veins: Limited Invaginated Axial Stripping and Tributary (hook) Stab Avulsion, *Ann Vasc Surg* 9 (1995): 401.

Chapter 5: Facial Spider Veins

1. JE Wenzl and EO Burgert, The Spider Nevus in Infancy and Childhood, *Pediatrics* 33 (1964): 227.

2. MP Goldman, *Sclerotherapy Treatment of Varicose and Telangiectatic Leg Veins* (St. Louis, Missouri: Mosby, 1995), 135.

3. MP Goldman et al, Treatment of Facial Telangiectasia with Sclerotherapy, Laser Surgery, and/or Electrodessication: A Review, *J Dermatol Surg Oncol* 19 (1993): 899.

4. ESC Medical Systems, Can Purpura Be Prevented When Treating Benign Vascular Lesions? (Needham, MA: ESC Medical Systems application notes, vol 1 no 1, 1996).

Chapter 6: Leg Vein Blood Clots

1. WW Coon, PW Willis III, and JB Keller, Venous Thromboembolism and Other Venous Disease in the Tecumseh Community Health Study, *Circulation* 48 (1973): 839.

2. J Ligush Jr and G Johnson Jr, Superficial Thrombophlebitis, in P Glovicki and JST Yao, *Handbook of Venous Disorders* (London: Chapman and Hall, 1996), 235.

3. HC Baron and BA Ross, *Varicose Veins: A Guide to Prevention and Treatment* (New York: Facts on File, Inc. 1995), 53.

4. EA Edwards, Thrombophlebitis of Varicose Veins, *Gynecol Obstet* 60 91938): 236.

5. JE Gjores, Surgical Therapy of Ascending Thrombophlebitis in the Saphenous System, *Angiology* 13 (1962): 241.

6. H Dodd and FB Cockett, *The Pathology and Surgery of the Lower Limb* (London: Churchill, Livingstone, 1976).

7. GHB Lewis and JF Hecker, Infusion thrombophlebitis, *Br J Anaesth* 57 (1985): 220.

8. MP Goldman, *Sclerotherapy Treatment of Varicose and Telangiectatic Leg Veins* (St. Louis, Missouri: Mosby, 1995), 69.

9. EA Husni and WA Williams, Superficial Thrombophlebitis of the Lower Limbs, *Surgery* 91 (1982): 70.

10. JM Lohr et al, Operative Management of Greater Saphenous Thrombophlebitis Involving the Sapheno-Femoral Junction, *Am J Surg* 164 (1992): 269.

11. G Goren, *Office Phlebology: A Practitioner's Guide* (Encino, CA: Nerog-Hill Desktop Publishing, 1995), 198.

12. E Ferrari et al, Travel as a Risk Factor in Venous Thrombotic Disease, *Chest* 112 (1997): 6S. (abstract)

13. S Conti, M Daschbach, and FW Blaisdell, A Comparison of High-Dose versus Conventional Dose Therapy for Deep Vein Thrombosis, *Surgery* 92 (1982): 972.

14. RD Hull et al, Continuous Infusion Heparin Compared with Intermittent Subcutaneous Heparin in the Initial Treatment of Proximal-Vein Thrombosis, *N Engl J Med* 315 (1986): 1109.

15. CS Landefeld et al, Identification and Preliminary Validation of Predictors of Major Bleeding in Hospitalized Patients Starting Anticoagulant Therapy, *Am J Med* 82 (1987): 703

16. AJ Comerota, Acute Deep Venous Thrombosis, in P Glovicki and JST Yao, *Handbook of Venous Disorders* (London: Chapman and Hall, 1996), 243.

17. MS Elliot et al, A Comparative Randomized Trial of Heparin versus Streptokinase in the Treatment of Acute Proximal Venous Thrombosis: An Interim Report of a Prospective Trial, *Br J Surg* 66 (1979): 838.

18. H Arnesen, A Hoiseth, and B Ly, Streptokinase or Heparin in the Treatment of Deep Vein Thrombosis: Follow-Up Results of a Prospective Study, *Acta Med Scand* 211 (1982): 65.

19. G Plate et al, Thrombectomy with Temporary Arteriovenous Fistula in Acute Iliofemoral Venous Thrombosis, *J Vasc Surg* 1 (1984): 867.

20. B Eklof and C Juhan, Revival of Thrombectomy in the Management of Acute Iliofemoral Venous Thrombosis, *Contemp Surg* 40 (1992): 21.

21. C Giuntini et al, Epidemiology, *Chest* 107 (1995): 3S.

22. HB Wheeler and FA Anderson Jr, Pulmonary Embolism, in P Glovicki and JST Yao, *Handbook of Venous Disorders* (London: Chapman and Hall, 1996), 274.

23. PD Stein, Deep Venous Thrombosis and Pulmonary Embolism, in the American College of Chest Physicians, *1997 Annual Scientific Assembly-Symposia Highlights* (American College of Chest Physicians, 1997), 4.

24. M Huisman et al, Unexpected High Prevalence of Pulmonary Embolism in Patients with Deep Venous Thrombosis, *Chest* 95 (1989): 498.

25. S Sevitt and N Gallagher, Venous Thrombosis and Pulmonary Embolism: A Clinico-Pathologic Study in Injured and Burned Patients, *Br J Surg* 45 (1961): 475.

26. JA Heit, Current Recommendations for Prevention of Deep Venous Thrombosis, in P Glovicki and JST Yao, *Handbook of Venous Disorders* (London: Chapman and Hall, 1996), 292.

27. C Lagerstedt et al, Need for Long-Term Anticoagulation Treatment in Symptomatic Calf-Vein Thrombosis, *Lancet* 2 (1989): 515.

28. PG Borozan et al, Non-invasive Imaging for Deep Venous Thrombosis, *Amer J Surg* 156 (1988): 474.

29. LJ Greenfield and MC Proctor, Indications and Techniques of Inferior Vena Cava Interruption, in P Glovicki and JST Yao, *Handbook of Venous Disorders* (London: Chapman and Hall, 1996), 306.

Chapter 7: The Swollen Leg

1. G Goren, *Office Phlebology: A Practitioner's Guide* (Encino, CA: Nerog-Hill Desktop Publishing, 1995), pg 202.

2. CS McEnroe, TF O'Donnell Jr, and WC Mackey, Correlation of Clinical Findings with Venous Hemodynamics in 386 Patients with Chronic Venous Insufficiency, *Am J Surg* 156 (1988): 148.

3. P Neglan and S Raju, A Rational Approach to Detection of Significant Reflux with Duplex Doppler Scanning and Air Plethysmography, *J Vasc Surg* 17 (1993): 590.

4. SK Shami et al, Venous Ulcers and the Superficial Venous System, *J Vasc Surg* 17 (1993): 487.

5. NM Wilson and NL Browse, Venous Disease, in DL Clement and JT Shepherd, ed, *Vascular Diseases in the Lower Limbs,* (St. Louis: 1993, Mosby Yearbook).

6. N Angle and JJ Bergan, Varicose Veins: Chronic Venous Insufficiency, in WS Moore, ed, *Vascular Surgery* (Philadelphia, 1997, WB Saunders Company), 800.

7. NL Browse and KG Burnand, The Postphlebitic Syndrome: A New Look, in JJ Bergan and JST Yao, *Venous Problems* (Chicago: Yearbook, 1978).

8. O Nelzen, D Bergqvist, and A Lindhagen, The Prevalence of Chronic Lower-Limb Ulceration has been Underestimated: Results of a Validated Population Questionaire, *Br J Surg* 83 (1996): 255.

9. P Glovicki and JST Yao, *Handbook of Venous Disorders* (London: Chapman and Hall, 1996), pg xv.

10. MP Goldman, *Sclerotherapy Treatment of Varicose and Telangiectatic Leg Veins* (St. Louis, Missouri: Mosby, 1995), 58.

11. MP Goldman, *Sclerotherapy Treatment of Varicose and Telangiectatic Leg Veins* (St. Louis, Missouri: Mosby, 1995), 64.

12. M Hume, Venous Ulcers, the Vascular Surgeon, and the Medicare Budget, *J Vasc Surg* 16 (1992): 671673.

13. CO Netzer and G Rudofsky, *Practical Ambulatory Phlebology* (Garching Near Munich, Germany: Verlag Medical Concept GmbH, 1991), 31.

14. MR Nehler, GL Moneta, and JM Porter, Nonoperative Management of Chronic Venous Insufficiency of the Lower Extremities, in P Glovicki and JST Yao, *Handbook of Venous Disorders* (London: Chapman and Hall, 1996), 416.

15. RG DePalma, Management of Incompetant Perforators: Conventional Techniques, in P Glovicki and JST Yao, *Handbook of Venous Disorders* (London: Chapman and Hall, 1996), 479.

Chapter 8: Arm Vein Blood Clots

1. T Holzenbein et al, Therapy and the Natural Course of Axillary Vein Thrombosis: Review of 765 Patients and Analysis of our Personal Patient Sample, *Vasa* Suppl 33 (1991): 107.

2. P Glovicki, RJ Kazmier, and LH Hollier, Axillary Subclavian Venous Occlusion: The Morbidity of a Nonlethal Disease, *J Vasc Surg* 4 (1986): 333.

3. NL Tilney, HFG Griffiths, and EA Edwards, Natural History of Major Venous Thrombosis of the Upper Extremity, *Arch Surg* 101 (1970): 792.

4. JA DeWeese, JT Adams , and DI Gaiser, Subclavian Venous Thrombectomy, *Circulation* 16 Suppl 2 (1970): 158.

5. RM Green, Acute Axillary-Subclavian Venous Thrombosis: Is Aggressive Management Justified? in P Glovicki and JST Yao, *Handbook of Venous Disorders* (London: Chapman and Hall, 1996), 260.

6. B Ardalan and MR Flores, A New Complication of Chemotherapy Administered via Permanent Indwelling Central Venous Catheter, *Cancer* 75 (1995): 2165.

7. B Brismar, C Hardstedt, and S Jacobson, Diagnosis of Thrombosis by Catheter Phlebography after Prolonged Central Venous Catheterization, *Ann Surg* 194 (1981): 779.

8. A Hingorani et al, Upper Extremity versus Lower Extremity Deep Vein Thrombosis, *Am J Surg* 174 (1997): 214.

Chapter 9: Don't Worry

1. Steadman's Medical, 23rd Edition, (Baltimore: The Williams and Wilkins Company, 1976).

2. J Theodosakis, B Adderlyand, and B Fox, *The Arthritis Cure* (New York: St. Martin's Paperbacks, 1997), 175.

Chapter 10: What You Can Do to Help Yourself

1. HC Baron and BA Ross, *Varicose Veins: A Guide To Prevention And Treatment* (New York: Facts on File, Inc. 1995), 30.

2. TL Cleave, *On Causation of Varicose Veins* (Bristol, United Kingdom: John Wright and Sons Ltd. 1960).

3. HC Baron and BA Ross, *Varicose Veins: A Guide to Prevention and Treatment* (New York: Facts on File, Inc. 1995), 91.

4. HC Baron and BA Ross, *Varicose Veins: A Guide to Prevention and Treatment* (New York: Facts on File, Inc. 1995), 75.

5. JA Heit, Current Recommendations for Prevention of Deep Venous Thrombosis, in P Glovicki and JST Yao, *Handbook of Venous Disorders* (London: Chapman and Hall, 1996), 292.

6. J Theodosakis, B Adderlyand, and B Fox, *The Arthritis Cure* (New York: St. Martin's Paperbacks, 1997), 113.

7. E Ferrari et al, Travel as a Risk Factor in Venous Thrombotic Disease, *Chest* 112 (1997): 6S. (abstract)

8. HC Baron and BA Ross, *Varicose Veins: A Guide to Prevention and Treatment* (New York: Facts on File, Inc. 1995), 99.

9. SL Malhotra, An Epidemiologic Study of Varicose Veins in Indian Railroad Workers from the South and North of India, with Special Reference to the Causation and Prevention of Varicose Veins, *Int J Epidemiol* 1 (1982): 117.

10. WE Connor, JG Hoak, and EA Warner, Massive Thrombosis Produced by Fatty Acid Infusion, *J Clin Invest* 42 (1963): 860.

11. WE Connor and JCF Poole, The Effect of Fatty Acids on the Formation of Thrombi, *Q J Exp Physiol* 46 (1961): 1.

12. JCF Poole, Effective Diet and Lipidemia on Coagulation and Thrombosis, *Fed Proc* 21 (1962): 20.

13. J Ludbrook, Obesity and Varicose Veins, *Surg Gynecol Obstet* 118 (1964): 843.

14. HP Wright and SB Osborn, Effect of Posture on Venous Velocity, *Br Heart J* 14 (1952): 325.

15. RSF Schilling and J Walford, Varicose Veins in Women Cotton Workers: an Epidemiologic Study in England and Egypt, *Br Med J* 2 (1969): 591.

Chapter 11: What's on the Horizon?

1. DM Duffy, Small Vessel Sclerotherapy: An Overview, *Adv Dermatol* 3 (1988): 221.

2. HC Baron and BA Ross, *Varicose Veins: A Guide to Prevention and Treatment* (New York: Facts on File, Inc. 1995), 23.

3. RL Kistner et al, The Evolving Management of Varicose Veins, *Postgrad Med* 80 (1986): 51.

4. K Biegeleisen and RD Nielsen, Failure of Angioscopically Guided Sclerotherapy to Permanently Obliterate Greater Saphenous Varicosity, *Phlebology* 9 (1994): 21.

5. JT Hobbs, Surgery and Sclerotherapy in the Treatment of Varicose Veins, *Arch Surg* 190 (1974): 793.

6. E Einarsson, B Eklof, and P Neglan, Sclerotherapy or Surgery as Treatment for Varicose Veins: A Prospective Randomized Study, *Phlebology* 8 (1993): 22.

7. CCR Bishop et al, Realtime Color Duplex Scanning After Sclerotherapy of the Greater Saphenous Vein, *J Vasc Surg* 14 (1991): 505.

8. A Gongolo et al, Il Sistema Duplex nel Follow-Up della Terapia Sclerosante della Vena Grande Saphena, *Radiol Med* (Italy) 81 (1991): 303.

9. C Legnani et al, Comparison of New Rapid Methods for D-dimer Measurement to Exclude Deep Vein Thrombosis in Symptomatic Outpatients, *Blood Coagul Fibrinolysis* 8 (1997): 296.

10. M Janssen et al, D-dimer Determination to Assess Regression of Deep Venous Thrombosis, *Thromb Haemost* 78 (1997): 799.

11. R Hull et al, Treatment of Proximal Vein Thrombosis with Subcutaneous Low-Molecular-Weight Heparin versus Intravenous Heparin: An Economic Perspective, *Arch Int Med* 157 (1997): 289.

12. G Goren, *Office Phlebology: A Practitioner's Guide* (Encino, CA: Nerog-Hill Desktop Publishing, 1995), 202.

13. CS McEnroe, TF O'Donnell Jr, and WC Mackey, Correlation of Clinical Findings with Venous Hemodynamics in 386 Patients with Chronic Venous Insufficiency, *Am J Surg* 156 (1988): 148.

14. P Neglan and S Raju, A Rational Approach to Detection of Significant Reflux with Duplex Doppler Scanning and Air Plethysmography, *J Vasc Surg* 17 (1993): 590.

15. SK Shami et al, Venous Ulcers and the Superficial Venous System, *J Vasc Surg* 17 (1993): 487.

16. NM Wilson and NL Browse, Venous Disease, in DL Clement and JT Shepherd, ed, *Vascular Diseases in the Lower Limbs* (St. Louis: Mosby Yearbook, 1993).

17. AA Rodriguez and TF O'Donnell Jr, Reconstructions for Valvular Incompetence of the Deep Veins, in P Glovicki and JST Yao, *Handbook of Venous Disorders* (London: Chapman and Hall, 1996), 434.

18. RG DePalma, Management of Incompetent Perforators: Conventional Techniques, in P Glovicki and JST Yao, *Handbook of Venous Disorders* (London: Chapman and Hall, 1996), 471.

19. TR Sullivan Jr and TF O'Donnell, Endoscopic Division of Incompetent Perforating Veins, in P Glovicki and JST Yao, *Handbook of Venous Disorders* (London: Chapman and Hall, 1996), 482.

20. MR Nehler, GL Monetta, and JM Porter, Nonoperative Management of Chronic Venous Insufficiency of the Lower Extremities, in P Glovicki and JST Yao, *Handbook of Venous Disorders* (London: Chapman and Hall, 1996), 416.

Chapter 12: Commonly Asked Questions

1. J Troisier, Le Bayon: Etude Genetique des Varices, *Ann de Med* (France) 41 (1937): 30.

2. C Ottley, Heredity and Varicose Veins, *Br Med J* 1 (1934): 528.

3. K Biegeleisen and RD Nielsen, Failure of Angioscopically Guided Sclerotherapy to Permanently Obliterate Greater Saphenous Varicosity, *Phlebology* 9 (1994):21.

4. N Angle and JJ Bergan, Varicose Veins: Chronic Venous Insufficiency, in WS Moore, *Vascular Surgery: A Comprehensive Review* (Philadelphia: WB Saunders Company, 1997), 800.

5. HC Baron and BA Ross, *Varicose Veins: A Guide to Prevention and Treatment* (New York: Facts on File, Inc. 1995), 53.

6. NL Browse and KG Burnand, The Postphlebitic Syndrome: A New Look, in JJ Bergan and JST Yao, *Venous Problems* (Chicago: Yearbook, 1978).

GLOSSARY OF TERMS

The following terms are explained as they are used in this book. Reference to standard medical dictionaries will provide more detailed explanations.

ABDOMEN: the part of the body that lies between the chest and the pelvis.

ABNORMAL: deviating from the normal.

ABSORB: the ability to take up.

ACUTE: rapid or sudden.

ANATOMY: the study of the structures of the body.

ANEURYSM: an outpouching or dilation of a portion of a blood vessel wall.

ANGIOGRAPHY: an x-ray outline of the blood vessels obtained after an injection of a radiopaque substance into it.

ANKLE: the joint connecting the leg and foot.

ANTICOAGULANT: a medicine that prevents the blood from clotting.

AORTA: the main artery in the body that carries the blood from the heart to everywhere else.

ARTERIOLE: a small artery that ends in the capillaries.

ARTERY: a vessel that carries blood from the heart to the body.

ATRIA: the upper collecting chambers of the heart. There is a right and left atrium.

BYPASS: a surgical procedure that routes blood around an obstructed vein or artery using artificial graft material or human tissue.

CALF: the back of the leg below the knee.

CANALIZATION: opening a passageway through a clotted vein.

CANCER: a general term frequently used to indicate various types of malignant tumors.

CAPILLARY: a thin-walled blood vessel where oxygen exchange occurs with the tissues of the body.

CARBON DIOXIDE: the end-product of metabolism. It is a common gas in the atmosphere. Plants convert carbon dioxide into oxygen by photosynthesis.

CARCINOMA: the medical term for cancer.

CARDIAC: relating to the heart.

CARDIOVASCULAR: relating to the blood vessels in the heart.

CAUTERIZATION: the use of heat or electric current to burn something. It is usually used as a method to control bleeding.

CAVITY: a hollow area or space within a body.

CELL: a minute living structure that varies in form according to the function it performs.

CHARLIE HORSE: a slang term for muscle spasm.

CHRONIC: with a long-term duration.

CHRONIC VENOUS INSUFFICIENCY: a long-term incompetency or leakage in the venous system, often leading to chronic skin changes and occasionally ulcer formation.

CIRCULATION: the passage of blood from the heart throughout the body and its return from the tissues back to the heart.

CIRRHOSIS: a damaged liver, frequently associated with chronic alcoholism.

CLAUDICATION: a cramp-like pain in the leg attributable to "hardening of the arteries." The pain, usually in the calf, occurs during walking and is relieved with rest.

CLINICAL: relating to the symptoms and course of a disease.

CLOT: a coagulation of blood within a vessel.

COAGULATION: the formation of a clot.

COLLAGEN: a major component of connective tissue.

COMMUNICATING VEINS: synonymous with perforator veins. They are the veins that connect the deep veins with the superficial veins.

COMPRESSION STOCKINGS: elastic garments that provide graduated pressure to improve venous drainage. They are commonly used on the legs and occasionally on the arms.

CONGENITAL: existing before birth.

CONNECTIVE TISSUE: the tissue surrounding and holding together cells of the body.

CONTRACEPTIVE: a medical device or drug used to prevent pregnancy.

CORONARY: relating to the heart, usually stated in relationship to the blood vessels of the heart.

COUMARIN: a blood-thinning medicine. The generic name is warfarin sodium.

CRAMP: painful muscle contraction. This is often the first symptom of varicose veins.

CUTANEOUS: relating to the outer layer of the skin.

CYANOSIS: a blue or purplish discoloration of the skin, most commonly the result of insufficient oxygen in the blood.

DEEP VEINS: the veins running near the bone beneath the fascia connective tissue of the leg.

DEEP VEIN THROMBOSIS: a blood clot in the deep veins of the legs.

DEPRESSION: a medical condition associated with a sinking of spirits.

DERMATITIS: an inflammation of the skin.

DERMATOLOGIST: a physician that specializes in skin disorders.

DIAGNOSIS: the determination of the causes of a disease.

DIASTOLE: the relaxation phase of the heart when it fills with blood.

DISEASE: a disorder of body functions.

DOPPLER: a noninvasive sound wave device used to measure blood flow in arteries and veins.

DORSUM: the back of an organ or body part.

DUPLEX ULTRASOUND: like sonar, a more sophisticated doppler interrogation that sends back pictures rather than just sound waves.

DYSFUNCTION: abnormal function of an organ or blood vessel.

ECZEMA: an acute or chronic inflammatory condition of the skin, frequently associated with redness, crusting, and itching.

EDEMA: an accumulation of excessive fluid in the tissues.

EMBOLISM: an obstruction or occlusion of a blood vessel; a transported clot.

EMBOLUS: a plug composed of a detached blood clot that breaks off and moves through the bloodstream to another place.

ENDOTHELIUM: the cells that form the inner lining of blood vessels.

ESTROGEN: the female sex hormone manufactured primarily in the ovaries.

ETIOLOGY: the study of a cause of disease.

EXCISE: to cut out or resect.

EXPIRATION: to breath out.

EXTRAVASATE: to exude from or pass out of a blood vessel into the tissue.

FAMILIAL VARICOSE VEINS: a condition sometimes called primary varicose veins; this form of varicose veins is associated with a hereditary component.

FASCIA: a sheet of fibrous tissues that envelopes muscles.

FEMORAL VEIN: the major vein in the leg that gets blood from the deep popliteal vein and superficial saphenous vein to feed into the deep iliac veins in the pelvis.

FEMUR: thigh bone; the bone from the hip to the knee.

FEVER: an elevated body temperature, above 37°C or 98.6°F.

FIBRIN: a protein that helps form clots.

FIBULA: the smaller of the two leg bones, on the outside of the calf.

FISSURE: a narrow break in the skin.

FOOT: the terminal part of the leg.

GANGRENE: a necrosis of tissue due to inadequate blood supply.

GAUZE: a cotton cloth used for dressings and bandages.

GENE: the functional unit of heredity. There are thousands of genes on chromosomes that are responsible for passing on characteristics from parent to child.

GERM: a bacteria or microorganism commonly associated with disease, a slang term for this would be a "bug."

GROIN: this is known as the inguinal area; it is the area between the front of the thigh and the abdomen.

HEART: the hollow, muscular four-chambered organ that receives blood from the veins and propels it to the lungs and the rest of the body. There are two receiving chambers (atria) and two pumping chambers (ventricles).

HEMATOMA: a localized mass of extravasated blood that is completely confined within a space. This usually goes on to form a contained blood clot.

HEMOGLOBIN: the portion of the red blood cell involved in oxygen transport. This is also the pigmented portion of the red blood cell.

HEMORRHAGE: bleeding, especially if it is profuse.

HEPARIN: a medicine that prevents blood from clotting.

HEREDITY: transmitted from parent to offspring.

Hg: the chemical symbol for mercury.

HIP: The joint on either side of the pelvis connecting the waist to the thigh.

HISTORY: the portion of the medical examination listing the patient's symptoms according to a sequence of events.

HORMONE: a chemical substance formed in one part of the body and carried in the blood stream to another.

HYPER: a prefix meaning excessive.

HYPO: a prefix meaning too little.

ILIAC VEIN: a major pelvic vein that connects the leg veins to the inferior vena cava.

INDURATION: extremely firm or hard.

INFERIOR VENA CAVA: the main blood vessel draining the lower portion of the body including the legs, pelvis, and abdomen. It is formed by the union of the common iliac veins and carries the blood upward to drain into the right atrium of the heart.

INFLAMMATION: a pathologic process associated with rubor (redness), calor (heat or warmth), tumor (swelling), and dolor (pain).

INFUSION: the injection of a solution into a vein.

INGUINAL REGION: the lower part of the abdominal wall also known as the groin.

INJECTION: the introduction of a medicine or other substance into (most often) a vein.

INTERSTITIAL: related to spaces or interstices in any structure.

INTIMA: the innermost lining of an artery or vein.

ISCHEMIA: an inadequate blood supply to an organ or extremity due to a blood vessel blockage (mainly arterial narrowing).

LATERAL: to the side, the opposite of toward the midline.

LEUKOCYTES: the white blood cells.

LIGATION: tying off blood vessels during surgery.

LIGATURE: the material used for tying off a blood vessel.

LUMEN: the space in the interior of a tubal structure such as an artery or vein.

LYMPH: a clear transparent fluid that is collected from tissues throughout the body that flows in the lymphatic vessels. It is eventually added to the venous blood circulation.

LYMPHATIC: pertaining to the channels that transport the lymph.

LYMPHEDEMA: abnormal swelling of the limb caused by the body's inability to drain the lymph channels.

MALIGNANT: resistant to treatment; tending to become worse and lead to a poor course.

MALLEOLUS: rounded bony prominences on either side of the ankle.

MELANIN: the brown pigmentation of the skin.

MELANOCYTES: the pigment cells containing melanin.

MEMBRANE: a thin sheet or layer of pliable tissue that covers or divides an organ.

MENOPAUSE: a permanent cessation of a woman's menstrual periods, commonly known as "the change of life."

MENSTRUAL PERIOD: the periodic, often monthly, discharge of bloody fluid by a woman from the uterus.

MILK LEG: the common name referring to an attack of phlebitis associated with a swollen leg that occurs with pregnancy.

MM: millimeter.

NECROSIS: the death of tissue most often due to inadequate blood supply.

OBESITY: an excessive accumulation of fat in the body; also known as "being overweight."

OBLITERATE: to close off.

OPERABLE: surgery can cause benefit.

ORGAN: a body part that performs a specific function.

OSTEOMYELITIS: an infection involving the bone.

PATENT: wide open.

PERFORATING VEINS: communicating veins that connect the superficial veins with the deep veins. These veins penetrate through the fascia and have valves that control the direction of blood flow. They are also often used to describe varicosities involving the veins on the lateral side of the calves.

PERIMENOPAUSAL: involving the early stages of menopause.

PERIPHERAL: relating to the outer part.

PHLEBECTOMY: the surgical excision of a portion of a vein.

PHLEBITIS: an inflammation of a vein.

PIGMENTATION: discoloration, either normal or abnormal, of the skin or tissues by a deposit, such as the red blood cells that stain into a brown discoloration related to varicosities around the ankle.

PLACEBO: an ineffective medicine given for its suggestive effects.

PLASMA: the fluid portion of the blood.

PLATELET: a very small blood component that plays a major role in blood clotting.

POLIDOCANOL: a commonly used sclerotherapy agent.

POPLITEAL VEIN: the deep vein that runs behind the knee bringing blood from the lower leg to the thigh.

PORT-WINE STAINS: a variation of spider veins, they most often appear on the face and neck as a very dense cluster of veins.

POSTERIOR: situated in the back of an organ.

POSTOPERATIVE: the time following a surgical procedure.

PROGESTERONE: a female hormone produced primarily by the ovaries.

PROPHYLAXIS: a measure carried out to prevent a disease.

PROSTHESIS: an artificial body part.

PROTEIN: a nutrient found in animal tissue.

PULMONARY CIRCULATION: the blood flow to and from the lungs where oxygen exchange occurs.

PULMONARY EMBOLISM: a blood clot lodged in the blood vessel to the lung. The clot usually originates from a broken off piece of a lower extremity deep vein clot. It is frequently fatal.

PURPURA: a very dense bruise caused by bleeding into the skin. It can be the result of some lasers.

RECANALIZATION: the natural reopening of a blocked blood vessel. This most often refers to a blood vessel reopening following a blood clot.

RETROGRADE: movement in the opposite direction of normal.

SALINE: a drug commonly used by doctors in sclerotherapy.

SAPHENOUS VEIN: a superficial leg vein that drains blood from the leg. The greater saphenous vein runs from the foot to the groin. It is the longest vein in the body. The lesser saphenous vein starts on the outside of the ankle and runs up the back of the calf to drain into the popliteal vein behind the knee.

SCLEROTHERAPY: the injection of a "hardening solution" into a vein to cause it to scar and obliterate. This is commonly used to treat spider veins.

SEQUELAE: the morbid condition following as a consequence of a disease.

SIGN: the physical evidence of a disease.

SOTRADECOL: a drug commonly used by doctors in sclerotherapy.

SPIDER VEINS: a cluster of dilated veins on the surface of the face, legs, and feet that are treated for symptoms or cosmetic reasons.

STRIPPING: a surgical procedure used to completely remove large segments of varicose veins.

SUBCUTANEOUS: beneath the skin.

SUPERFICIAL: obtaining to the surface.

SUPERFICIAL VEINS: the veins situated just beneath the skin in the subcutaneous fatty tissue, including the greater and lesser saphenous veins of the legs.

SUPERIOR: the highest part of an organ or body.

SUPERIOR VENA CAVA: the main blood vessel draining the upper part of the body including the head, arms, and chest. It is formed by the union of several veins and carries the blood into the right atrium of the heart.

SYMPTOM: a sign or evidence of departure from a normal condition.

SYNDROME: a group of signs and symptoms that form a pattern of disease.

SYSTEMIC: a) the blood flow throughout the body except for the pulmonary circulation, b) a condition involving the entire body.

SYSTOLE: the contraction phase of the heart, which pumps the blood throughout the body.

TELANGIECTASIAS: the dilation and stretching of small or terminal blood vessels. These are usually reddish-purple discolored spider veins.

THERAPY: the treatment of an illness or disorder.

THROMBECTOMY: the surgical removal of a blood clot that is obstructing a blood vessel.

THROMBOPHLEBITIS: an inflamed vein with secondary blood clot formation.

THROMBOSIS: the formation of a blood clot in a blood vessel.

TISSUE: a grouping of cells of a similar type.

TORTUOUS: many twist and turns.

ULCER: a pitted sore on the surface of the skin.

UNILATERAL: affecting only one side of the body.

UNNA BOOT: a wrap of medicated bandages that solidifies into a cast-like material. It is used to help venous ulcers heal.

VALSALVA MANEUVER: a maneuver where patients hold their breath and bear down, causing an increase in the blood pressure of the abdomen, which is then transferred into an increase in venous blood pressure in the lower extremities. This technique is used to look for malfunctioning vein valves in the legs.

VALVE: a one-way opening in veins that keeps the blood flowing in the proper direction from the body back to the heart.

VARICOSE: an enlarged and tortuous vein.

VARICOSITIES: multiple dilated and tortuous veins, usually referring to the superficial saphenous veins of the legs and their branches.

VARIX: the term for a single dilated vein.

VARICOSE ULCER: skin breakdown in the drainage area of a varicose vein, usually just above the ankle, resulting from stasis.

VASCULARIZATION: the formation of new blood vessels.

VEINS: the blood vessels that carry blood back to the heart from the remainder of the body.

VENA CAVAE: the two largest veins in the body. The inferior vena cava drains blood from the lower extremities and abdomen; the superior vena cava drains blood from the upper extremities and head to the heart.

VENOGRAM: an x-ray of a vein taken following injection of a thick substance to outline its course.

VENOUS STASIS: slow-flowing blood within a vein.

VENOUS STASIS ULCER: a skin breakdown that is the result of stagnant blood flow, often due to vein valve leakage.

VENTRICLES: the two pumping chambers of the heart, left and right.

VENULES: small draining veins that connect the larger veins to the capillaries, where oxygen exchange occurs.

WARFARIN: orally administered long-term blood-thinning medicine used to treat patients who have developed clots.

X-RAY: a picture taken of the body using electromagnetic radiation.

INDEX

INDEX

INDEX

INDEX

INDEX